Community Art Therapy

This book provides a narrative exploration of community art therapy woven from its rich practice roots, theory, the multiple ways that it can be applied in practice, and through practitioner reflections.

The applications of community art therapy are numerous, and this book provides knowledge to practitioners, guiding them in their own work and grounding their theoretical approaches. The community approaches presented in the text have been developed through careful research, strategy, and implementation.

Community Art Therapy is for the benefit of art therapists, community artists and psychologists, and anyone interested in learning more about the stories of community art therapy.

Emily Goldstein Nolan, DAT (she/her) is an art therapist and art therapy educator, professional counselor, and a professor of practice at Syracuse University. Her specialties include working with communities and those people who have experienced trauma.

Community Art Therapy

Theory and Practice

Emily Goldstein Nolan

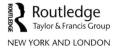

Routledge
Taylor & Francis Group

NEW YORK AND LONDON

Designed cover image by Emily Goldstein Nolan

First published 2024
by Routledge
605 Third Avenue, New York, NY 10158

and by Routledge
4 Park Square, Milton Park, Abingdon, Oxon, OX14 4RN

Routledge is an imprint of the Taylor & Francis Group, an informa business

Library of Congress Cataloging-in-Publication Data
Names: Nolan, Emily Goldstein, author.
Title: Community art therapy: theory and practice / by Emily Goldstein Nolan,
DAT, Syracuse University, Syracuse, NY.
Description: New York, NY: Routledge, 2024. | Includes bibliographical references and index. |
Identifiers: LCCN 2023009581 (print) | LCCN 2023009582 (ebook) |
ISBN 9781032044590 (hardback) | ISBN 9781032044583 (paperback) |
ISBN 9781003193289 (ebook)
Subjects: LCSH: Art therapy. | Artists and community. |
Community arts projects–Therapeutic use.
Classification: LCC RC489.A7 N65 2024 (print) | LCC RC489.A7 (ebook) |
DDC 616.89/1656–dc23/eng/20230527
LC record available at https://lccn.loc.gov/2023009581
LC ebook record available at https://lccn.loc.gov/2023009582

ISBN: 978-1-032-04459-0 (hbk)
ISBN: 978-1-032-04458-3 (pbk)
ISBN: 978-1-003-19328-9 (ebk)

DOI: 10.4324/9781003193289

Typeset in Times New Roman
by Deanta Global Publishing Services, Chennai, India

For Liam, Maisie, and Jasper.
You are loved.

Contents

Illustrations

Figures

Images

Contributing Authors

Pat B. Allen, PhD, ATR, (she/her) lives in Berkeley, CA, and Sarasota, FL. Her art therapy education began in the 1970s in an apprenticeship with Margaret Naumburg. She is a co-founder of the Open Studio Project and continues to teach and collaborate in bringing the Open Studio Process into more forms and forums around the world. Pat centers the artist identity in her work to activate the inherent creativity in all people. Her present work involves using the Open Studio Process to unpack and dismantle white supremacy and to explore and heal generational trauma. She is a senior educator at Jewish Studio Project, an enterprise founded by her daughter, Rabbi Adina Allen.

Thahmina Begum, BA (Hons), (she/her) is based in Yorkshire, United Kingdom. She is currently studying for her master's in art psychotherapy practice with the Northern Programme based at Sheffield Health and Care Trust and Leeds Beckett University. Thahmina has over 20 years' experience of community art projects with grassroots groups; her research interests are racial and intergenerational trauma, community art therapy and hyperlocal histories.

Erica Browne, ATR, LPC, (she/her) is an artist, art therapist, licensed professional counselor, and director at Bloom Art and Integrated Therapies, a community-based art therapy non-profit located in Milwaukee, Wisconsin. Through Bloom, Erica provides trauma-informed art therapy to underserved youth in the Milwaukee Public Schools as part of a restorative program in collaboration with Marquette University and other community mental health and wellness providers. Erica's artistic work explores the intersection of relational art, social practice, and art therapy.

Jennifer DeLucia, DAT, LCAT, (she/her) is an assistant professor and founding chair of the Department of Creative Arts Therapy at Syracuse University and is the curator of the University's National Veterans Resource Center art gallery. She lives in Rochester, New York, and has over 15 years of art therapy experience across outpatient, private practice, and community-based settings. DeLucia received her Doctorate in Art Therapy from Mount Mary University in Milwaukee, Wisconsin, USA.

Andrea Inés Velázquez Dorgan, MAAT, ATR (she/her) has had the opportunity to live in the United States, Switzerland, and, currently, Mexico City, thus having been able to experience art therapy with different populations and formats. She is founder of Open Studio Mexico, a project where the spirit of art and its medicine are explored and shared from Mexican and Latin American roots as a vehicle of change. Currently, she is reconnecting, recreating, and taking ownership of her childhood home.

Kai Ying Huang, DAT, ATR-BC (she/her) is based in northern Taiwan. She is an assistant professor in the University of Taipei Graduate Department of Visual Arts with specialized training in art therapy. She received her Master of Science in art therapy and counseling from the College of New Rochelle, in New York and her Doctorate in Art Therapy from Mount Mary University in Milwaukee, Wisconsin. Her work is dedicated to working with people who have experienced trauma in Asian communities.

Louvenia Jackson, PhD, LMFT, ATR-BC (she/her) is associate professor and chairperson at Loyola Marymount University Graduate Department of Marital Family Therapy with specialized training in art therapy. She received her MFT and PhD from Notre Dame de Namur University Art Therapy Psychology Department. Her work on cultural humility can be found in her first authored book, *Cultural Humility in Art Therapy: The Balance of Creativity, Introspection and Advocacy.*

Lynn Kapitan, PhD, ATR-BC, HLM, (she/her) is an art therapist, educator, and founder of the master's and doctoral art therapy programs at Mount Mary University in Milwaukee, WI, USA. She has worked with a wide variety of groups and people in alternative settings, and for the past 20 years has practiced community art therapy as a pro bono research consultant for a local non-governmental organization based in Managua, Nicaragua that promotes community-led projects for social transformation in urban and rural communities throughout the country.

Owen Karcher, MA, LPC, ATR-BC, (he/they) is an art therapist, lecturer, author, and social justice consultant. He works with the individual and collective healing of trauma and oppression through embodied, creative expression. Owen facilitates group processes that explore how power, privilege, and identities impact participants' relationships and work. He has 15 years of experience working in mental health, violence prevention and intervention, HIV/AIDS, building healthy relationships, LGBTQ resiliency, and organizing toward social justice.

Chelsea O'Neil, MA, ATR, (they/them) is an art therapist, social justice educator, and full-spectrum doula. Chelsea is currently pursuing an EdD in student affairs administration and leadership specializing in LGBTQ+ student development, liberatory social justice pedagogy, and the critical analysis of social inequities in higher education. As a scholar practitioner, Chelsea's work is dedicated to cultivating healing, hope, and opportunity for all people through systemic change and intentional relationship building.

Ling Cheun Bianca Lee, LCPC, LMHC, ATR-BC, (she/her) divides her time between Hong Kong and the United States. She is a private practitioner with a transnational practice and an educator/ supervisor for multiple universities. She obtained her Master of Art in art therapy from the School of the Art Institute of Chicago.

Lauren Leone, DAT, ATR-BC, LMHC, (she/her) lives in Somerville, Massachusetts where she works with art therapy participants in private and community-based settings. She received her Master of Arts in art therapy and mental health counseling from Lesley University in Cambridge, MA and her Doctorate in Art Therapy from Mount Mary University in Milwaukee, WI.

Angela Lyonsmith DAT, ATR-BC, ATCS, LCPC, (she/her) creates home with her family in Evanston, IL. Her passion for the intersection of art-making, community-building, and wellness is expressed through her professional work that spans art therapy practice and education. She earned her MA in Art Therapy at the School of the Art Institute of Chicago and her Doctoral degree at Mount Mary University. She is a founding director of Kids Create Change and Studio 3, where she offers children and families opportunities to access creativity while encouraging empathy, connection, and community care.

Abbe Miller, PhD, MS, ATR-BC, LPC, (she/her) is based in Connecticut, in the United States. She discovered the field of art therapy in the 1970s and has been loving the path that led her to create the El Duende method. Abbe has been a dedicated graduate program educator and continues to provide soulful art-based supervision and artistic discovery to nurture the emergence of authentic voice and to share it with those who come to her home-based studio/office.

Gretchen M. Miller, MA, ATR-BC, ACTP, (she/her) is a registered board-certified art therapist and advanced certified trauma practitioner who has been practicing in Northeast Ohio, United States for over 20 years. Her art therapy work has included youth and adults impacted by trauma and loss, academic teaching, supervision, and community organizing. Gretchen received her master's in art therapy from Ursuline College.

Melissa Raman Molitor, MA, ATR-BC, LCPC, (she/her) is an associate adjunct professor at the School of the Art Institute of Chicago where she received her MA in Art Therapy. She is a founding director of the non-profit organization Kids Create Change, working with young people to explore identity, engender empathy and care, and make change in the community through the arts. She is also the founder of the Kitchen Table Stories Project and Evanston ASAPIA providing art-based initiatives to increase the visibility and representation of the local Asian, South Asian, Pacific Islander American community through placemaking and storytelling.

Rachel K. Monaco, JD (she/her), works from Wisconsin, in the United States, dividing her time between the Milwaukee area and the South Shore of Lake Superior. She is the founder of LOTUS Legal Clinic, serving the legal needs of, and empowering, victims of sexual violence and human trafficking. She came to the field of art therapy through teaching in Mount Mary University's art therapy doctoral program as a multi-disciplinary professional in law, non-profits, restorative justice, victims' rights, and conflict resolution. She received her degrees in Law, English and Theology from Marquette University.

Dani Moss, DAT, ATR-BC, LPC, ATCS, NCC, (she/her) is an art therapist and counselor. She serves as assistant professor of art therapy and internship coordinator in the master's in art therapy with specialization in counseling program at Seton Hill University in Greensburg, Pennsylvania. Dani's professional art therapy experience includes clinical and community program development in many settings in multiple counties and states working with children, families, elders, and organizations. She currently teaches art therapy theory, research, internship courses, and advises theses.

Emily Goldstein Nolan, DAT, LCAT, LPC, ATR-BC, (she/her) is a professor of practice and practicum/internship coordinator at Syracuse University, a licensed professional counselor, and a licensed art psychotherapist. In 2012, she founded Bloom Art and Integrated Therapies, Inc, a community-based art therapy non-profit in Milwaukee, Wisconsin. Dr. Nolan is the founder of, and develops and oversees, the community art therapy programs for Bloom. Dr. Nolan is dedicated to educating art therapists and working with people who have experienced trauma and have been historically excluded to feel seen, heard, and understood.

Rochele Royster, PhD, ATR-BC, (she/her) originally from rural Virginia, has lived on the South Side of Chicago for the last 20 years. She has recently relocated to Syracuse, New York, in the United States to work as assistant professor in the Creative Art Therapy Department at Syracuse University. After obtaining a graduate degree in special education and realizing therapeutic skills were needed to understand, support, and address behaviors and emotional literacy in the classroom, she received her master's in art therapy from The School of the Art Institute of Chicago.

Laura Swift MS, LPC, ATR, (she/her) has called Milwaukee, Wisconsin, home for more than 17 years. She attended the graduate art therapy program at Mount Mary University where she has since been an instructor in both the graduate and undergraduate art therapy programs. She continues to specialize in serving adjudicated youth in Milwaukee, working passionately to create art-based opportunities to connect youth to the community.

Yasmin Tucker MS, LPC, ATR, (she /her) is the founder, owner, and chief executive officer of Creative Counseling and Studio in Omaha, Nebraska. Yasmin is a child, teen, and adult therapist who specializes in art therapy, EMDR, CPP, DBT, trauma-informed and multiculturally sensitive care. Yasmin provides individual therapy for people(s) of all ages and backgrounds. Yasmin is a nationally registered art therapist, licensed independent mental health practitioner, licensed professional counselor, and provisionally licensed alcohol and drug counselor. She has worked with children, adults, persons in recovery from substances, people struggling with severe and persistent mental illnesses, parent–child dyads, families, and couples.

Allison Tunis, BFA, DVATI, (she/they) works on Treaty 6 territory in Amiskwaciwâskahikan (Edmonton), Alberta, Canada. Working from both her education in fine arts (University of Alberta, 2008) and art therapy (Vancouver Art Therapy Institute, 2013), Allison focuses on using community arts to foster stronger and better-connected communities and individuals.

Research Contributors

I interviewed the following community practitioners for this book. Each person has given their permission to share their names and practice locations with readers.

Aleksic, Mina	Belgrade, Serbia
Alfonso, Gina	Manila, Philippines
Andrasikova, Karina	Bratislava, Slovakia
Arbeitman, Elissa	Manalapan, New Jersey
Baker, Sara	Pittsburgh, Pennsylvania
Begum, Thahmina	Leeds, United Kingdom
Belnavis Elliot, Lesli-Ann	Kingston, Jamaica
Byrne, Julia	Hong Kong, SAR, China
Chakrabarthi, Oihika	India; Kolkata, Mumbai, Sri Lanka
Donald, Karina	Grenada
Echeverry, María Cristina Ruiz	Cali, Colombia
Frazier, Steve	Mexico City, Mexico
García, Ana	Montréal, Canada
Glinzak, Leara	Aurora, Colorado
Goldstraw, Sally	Melbourne, Australia
Guyen, Linh	Vietnam
Jankovic Shentser, Mia	Croatia
Krüger, Carolyn	Berlin, Germany
Lee, Bianca	Hong Kong
Leung, Paisley	Hong Kong
Lopez, María Reyes	Bogotá, Colombia
Luzzatto, Paola	Italy/Tanzania
Mariño, Luisa	Maryland
Moon, Cathy	Chicago, Illinois
Myburgh, Rozanne	Johannesburg, South Africa

Ng, Jue Ann	Singapore
Orbach, Nona	Isreal
Siirtola, Anne	Karkkila, Finland
Ter Maat, Mercedes	Florida, Argentina
Volonts, Julia	Latvia; New York, New York
Whitaker, Pamela	Ireland
Yi, Sandie	Chicago, IL

Foreword

Community art practices have had an influence in the development of Western art therapy with examples of primarily women successfully using the arts to bolster and address complex needs in their own communities. It has been my experience that over the past 30 years the community aspect of art therapy has been operating quite well on the margins, safe from calcifying "specialization" definitions and credentialing considerations. This has provided freedom to grow, make necessary mistakes, and see what works for each project.

Emily Goldstein Nolan has taken a different approach, which I greatly appreciate. Simultaneous to her practice she set out to locate explanations and define community art therapy through a grounded theory lens. By inviting seasoned art therapists and other highly qualified voices from 36 different countries to contribute, she has written a compelling offering. I am thrilled that her definition, fueled by many voices, reflects the breadth and diversity of practices and their geographical contexts.

Pressing reasons for centering community art therapy within our profession are abundant but one urgent motive stands out. The chasm created by a lack of accessible mental health care services during and following the initial pandemic has had a profound negative effect in many communities. No one escaped the experience of mandated social isolation and the changes in access to families and friends. Things we formerly took for granted were lost. We now have further "proof" that as a population we require access to social environments that care for people's connections to each other. We experienced first-hand how the creative arts worked to help hold us together when we could no longer meet in our physical community studios. We were reminded again that we need to work to prioritize the inclusion of the creative arts in policies concerning our well-being to weather future storms.

In this text, art therapists and other creative arts practitioners from different global contexts offer their relevant and heart-felt community practice reflections as well as new ways of conceptualizing and theorizing community art therapy.

Based on extensive practitioner interviews, for example, a beehive model of community art therapy emerged, which bridges theory and practice. Another example is Rochele Royster's Salt of the Earth theory and practice welcoming a broader ecological perspective of research as a way of leveling the playing field. Colleagues, along with Emily Goldstein Nolan, share tools based on their experiences of developing and evaluating programs as well as educating, training, and supervising students. There is also an important discussion about ethical dilemmas that emerge outside the narrow confines of professional ethics.

Over the years sustained practices of many community art therapy projects and programs have had a quiet grassroots ripple effect and it is now time to give it its proper place in the profession many of us have devoted our careers to. Join me in congratulating Emily Goldstein Nolan, her collaborators, and all the interviewees for taking time from their practices to give us their generous expert perspectives.

Community art therapy is positioned to play a major role in a rapidly changing world. I hope you will join in this movement starting with this informative text. By listening carefully to each other and to the voices in our communities, we can tell our stories much like the authors of this book and put into action many small, dynamic, and sustainable solutions.

Janis Timm-Bottos, PhD, ATR-BC
Montreal, QC
Canada

Acknowledgments

This book marks the completion of a lifelong dream. From the time I was little, I found myself escaping to the library and getting lost in books. Once my mom showed me the way to the library, I was there all the time. Reading and education opened possibilities for me that I could have never imagined on my own. Through my love of books, I became fascinated with writing and how I might be able to share what I learn with others. Which is one more thing I love—exploring something new and then discussing what I find with other people.

This project is an act of community and this book's existence is not without the help and support of many others. I would like to thank all the therapists and community members who have ever worked with me in any version of Bloom—I have learned great things from all of you. I would like to thank the interview participants and reflection writers for contributing their stories and sharing their incredibly important work. Most of the reflections are contained within one chapter, but there are a few reflections that have been woven into the chapters. I am so very grateful for Rochele Royster's expertise in community psychology and research. Rochele read this book and shared her thoughts, insights, and encouragement throughout the process. My fantastic research assistant, Julia Mumpton, transcribed all the interviews, helped to triangulate findings, wrote the chapter abstracts, and her attention to detail is such a gift. Lynn Kapitan, my long-time research mentor, helped me with this project from the beginning and was essential in validating the findings and shaping the theory. Janis Timm-Bottos was instrumental in helping me refine my writing and ideas. Routledge provided me with a publishing platform, ample time to gather and analyze the interview data, and guided me through the process of book publication. Thank you to Chelsea Goldwell for designing the book cover and always being a supportive part of my community. Shannon Tasei designed the beautiful figures included in the book. Rachel Monaco has been an exceptional book doula, keeping me on task, and managing publishing details. She has been right there with me at each step, helping to reason through ideas and concepts that emerged in the data in a way that could be accessible to the reader.

Finally, my husband Sean has kept me grounded and hopeful as I often shared my worst fears about writing this book with him. He has an uncanny ability to challenge me and keep me centered, focused, and real. I love him for that.

Chapter 1

Introducing People, Places, Tools, and Processes in Community Art Therapy

Emily Goldstein Nolan

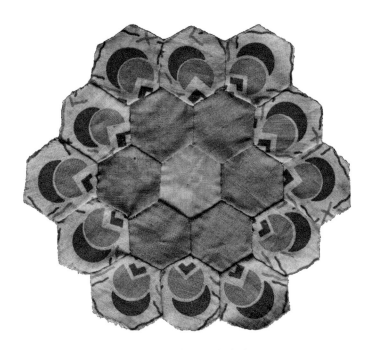

Honeycomb quilt block 1

Introduction

Part of the impetus for writing this book was that I sought a clear definition of community art therapy. I began integrating intentional community practices into my work as an art therapist in 2011. I searched for articles and examples that discussed the development of community art therapy at that time to include in my dissertation literature review and inform my practice. I wondered why no one had defined community art therapy before; I thought maybe it had something to do

DOI: 10.4324/9781003193289-1

with the historical binary discussions of artist or therapist, art psychotherapy or art as therapy, and the fear that art therapists were moving toward "clinification" of the field (Allen, 1992). Maybe, I considered, art therapists shied away from discussing community endeavors to justify the field and promote acceptance as a legitimate treatment, art therapists as equals in collaboration with other mental health treatment providers, and for gaining credentials and licensing. Many research and subsequent publications in the last ten years do explicate aspects of community art therapy practice. And since then, the space continues to ripen for a definition of community art therapy. However, as I began the research to write this book, it was evident very early on that community art therapy has not been defined in large part *because it looks different depending on where it is practiced and how the offerings are created and implemented.* Defining community art therapy potentially flattens the richness that encompasses the people, tools, processes, strengths, and challenges that comprise it. Multitudes of community art therapy practices exist and any one way to practice is definitely not the *right* way for every setting. Community art therapy emerges from and within the cultures and contexts in which it occurs; it is alive and ever evolving. However, although it is contextual and culturally practiced in its served population and geographical setting, there are important common approaches that professionals can use to focus their own practices. My vision for this book is that it provides a guide for community practices in art therapy based on the stories, experiences, and knowledge of art therapy practitioners who are deep in the work.

One Size Does Not Fit All

A theory of community art therapy begins with considering how a community is distinguished. For the purposes of this book, the community is an aggregate of people with a shared interest and location to one another (Ritter & Lampkin, 2012). Using the language of mental health treatment, the client is the consumer of therapy services. In family therapy there may be an individual within the family who is the identified client. In group therapy the group is the client. Therefore, from a community mental health conceptualization, the community is considered the client. Subsequent chapters of this book that discuss the theory and practice deconstruct the notion of client, and participants, as well as who and what types of groups can be considered a community.

An additional important step toward theory is defining community art therapy. Interestingly, when interviewing many of the art therapists who have had vast experiences of art therapy practice to draw from, they were naturally concerned about how I would define community art therapy. From the interviews and reflections within this text the following definition emerged:

> Community art therapy is both an approach and a setting, defined in the context of the culture that it is practiced in through an intention shared by those

trained in art therapy practice with a group of people who have a collective interest in art making as a transformative and therapeutic process.

To some, culture itself is contextual and resists deductive definitions (Jahoda, 2012). However, it is also important to define culture as it is used here. I conceptualized culture considering that "is a multidimensional phenomenon that encompasses processes, products and results of human activity, material and spiritual" (Mironenko & Sorokin, 2018, p. 338), and it is passed on from generation to generation.

From Definition to Theory

The broad definition presented of community art therapy leaves space to contextualize the practice and discuss the common factors in the aims that are present within the experiences of each setting explored. Pluralism is a theory positing that multiple truths exist within one defined setting (Kaul & Salvatore, 2020). If art therapy is the setting, then the practice of art therapy can be varied and all the ways that it transpires can coexist. Salom (2017) wrote, "by claiming and carrying the polarity within our practices," art therapists can change "research and platforms for dialogue, new diagnostic understanding for a pluralistic society, and treatment modalities that can be analyzed both inside and outside the limitations of Western constructs" (p. 73). Art therapy is practiced in countries all over the world. Effective diverse practices are not extrapolated from the United States and the UK; at best, world practices can mutually influence one another (Kalmanowitz et al., 2009, p. 318). World practices of art therapy exist and have developed uniquely to the geographical area in which they are taking place. As community art therapy exists and emerges everywhere, practitioners have an incredible opportunity to share what they have learned with each other.

I have practiced community art therapy mostly in the midwestern and eastern portions of the United States. Rather than define community art therapy and write a book based on that one experience of practice, I have sought to construct a theory "grounded" in the data of many other creative practitioner experiences (Charmaz, 2014). For me, contributing a grounded theory and model of community art therapy embraces the ideal that it is viewed as whole, dynamic, and continuously changing and adapting.

Organization of the Book by Chapter

In the following pages I discuss the definition of community art therapy that emerged from interviewing practitioners and lay out the people, places, processes, and tools that comprise its practice. Practice examples of community art therapy include 36 different countries with information from 32 practitioner interviews. The research conducted to develop grounded theory from interviews received Internal Review Board exempt approval through Syracuse University.

In Chapter 2, I explicate and discuss the grounded theory of the definition and practitioners approaches to community art therapy. I provide further foundation for the theory with integrated literature sources that have informed the practice of community art therapy. This chapter also presents a beehive model of community art therapy that bridges theory and practice.

In Chapter 3, art therapists who practice in community contexts all over the world contribute reflections that shed light on their projects and organizations. These contributions give voice to the important work happening in community art therapy, inspiring other art therapists and community workers.

In Chapter 4, I discuss considerations for the education and supervision of art therapists who work in community contexts. Erica Browne and Yasmin Tucker provide a reflection on their experiences of supervision in the community through the lens of both the supervisor and the intern.

In Chapter 5, I present information about developing and evaluating community art therapy programs. This chapter provides action research as a tool art therapists can use to develop, implement, and evaluate their own programs. Rachel Monaco contributes a reflection about the development and evaluation of the Untold Stories project with survivors of sex trafficking.

In Chapter 6, I explore challenges and ethical dilemmas that art therapists grapple with when working in community art therapy endeavors. Kaiying Huang provides a reflection based on her experiences of being a sojourner art therapist trained in the United States but practicing in Taiwan. Her reflection explores the ethical considerations she sees as necessary when trained outside of the geographical location and culture where she practices.

In Chapter 7, I present ideals for engaging in embodied community art therapy research and discuss challenges of community research. In her reflection, Rochele Royster offers her experiences and considerations for working with communities.

In Chapter 8, I conclude by summarizing key points from the book and asking some further questions that have emerged for me during the researching and writing of this book.

Limitations and Considerations

It is important to note that this book, while primarily written by one author, has many contributors. I understand that my white, middle-class, cisgender female lens is limited, and it is only through collaboration with the contributing authors and practitioners who dedicated their time, experiences, and their stories that I can present this text. Additionally, as I have searched the literature, I found that most historical information about the development of art therapy is held by the United States and the UK, with some information from Asia and Australia. When I saw how little information I could find in the literature representing the many countries where community art therapy happens, I had the desire and felt a responsibility to interview art therapists practicing all over the world. In doing so, I am not taking on the role of art therapy historian. Documenting a timeline of the history of community art therapy potentially runs the risk of privileging whose story gets told and whose gets left out. I know that I am limited by my perspective and by where I practice community art therapy. Many historical examples and ancestors of community art therapy practice exist, but it is not within the scope of this text to explore every one of them. In part, this is due to the lack of access to information: Some projects and efforts have been recorded locally or not at all. The incomplete and tremendous task of telling a global history or complete story acknowledges that some published works are written in languages I do not speak or read. Additionally, when interviewing art therapists, I am limited by my ability to speak only English. I chose not to use interpreters due to high costs and publishing time constraints. I conducted the interviews over an online video communication platform. The advent of the coronavirus pandemic made many technologies for this type of communication widely available, but there were still folks I was not able to interview because they did not have the technology available to them. Additionally, I use the terms art therapist and art therapy practitioner interchangeably throughout the text. Not all people working in community are formally educated art therapists due to emerging art therapy infrastructures in many geographical locations and lack of access to university training.

Conclusion

My hope is that what I share here will adequately situate current theories and practices of community art therapy, by giving attention to, and sharing, the multiple pathways along which it can be implemented. I have had the very special gift of speaking with art and creative therapists and practitioners in many different geographical locations from many different racial, ethnic, socioeconomic, and cultural backgrounds. What I have learned is that community art therapy has developed out of a rich expanse of people who were and are deeply engaged in not only the creative process but also the health and long-term well-being of those in the communities around them.

References

Allen, P. (1992). Artist in residence: An alternative to "clinification" for art therapists. *Art Therapy*, *9*(1), 22–29. https://doi.org/10.1080/07421656.1992.10758933

Charmaz, K. (2014). *Constructing grounded theory* (2nd ed.). Sage.

Jahoda, G. (2012). Critical reflections on some recent definitions of "culture". *Culture and Psychology*, *18*(3), 289–303. https://doi.org/10.1177/1354067X12446229

Kalmanowitz, D., Potash, J., & Chan, S. M. (Eds.). (2009). *Art therapy in Asia: To the bone or wrapped in silk*. Jessica Kingsley.

Kaul, V., & Salvatore, I. (Eds.). (2020). *What is pluralism?* Routledge. https://doi-org
.libezproxy2.syr.edu/10.4324/9780367814496

Mironenko, I., & Sorokin, P. (2018). Seeking for the definition of "culture": Current
concerns and their implications. A comment on Gustav Jahoda's article "critical
reflections on some recent definitions of 'culture'". *Integrative Psychological
Behavior*, *52*(2), 331–340. https://doi.org /10.1007/s12124-018-9425-y

Ritter, L., & Lampkin, S. (2012). *Community mental health*. Jones and Barlett learning.

Salom, A. (2017). Claiming polarity in art therapy: Lessons from the field in Columbia.
Art Therapy, *34*(2), 68–74. https://doi.org/10.1080/07421656.2017.1312152

Chapter 2

Community Art Therapy and its Approaches

Emily Goldstein Nolan

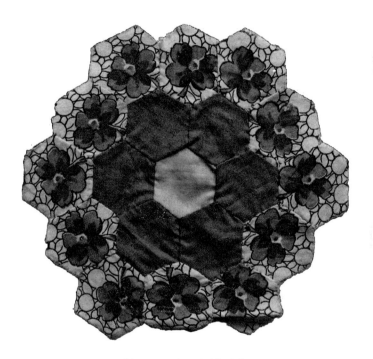

Honeycomb quilt block 2

Introduction

The purpose of this chapter is to present theory defining community art therapy and practitioner methods. From theory, I created a model of community art therapy. The intention is that this model will guide art therapists working in community approaches and settings.

DOI: 10.4324/9781003193289-2

Background

The theory presented here has a few key underpinnings that are important to keep in mind. In this text, community is defined as a group of people who gather around a specific purpose or interest. Additionally, community art therapy is defined as an approach and a setting influenced by the context of the culture that it is practiced in, through an intention shared by those trained in art therapy practice, with a group of people who have a collective interest in artmaking as a transformative and therapeutic process.

Community art therapy has been evolving since the art therapy field first developed in the early 20th century. The literature on art therapy tells the story of art therapy's growth so far, and how art therapists often struggled with identity and how to define art therapy. Art therapists in current practice know that they are both, artists and therapists, without a need to tether themselves to one identity and can pull from a spectrum of practice approaches (Vick, 1996; Potash et al., 2016). However, reading about community art therapy endeavors in the literature as it has unfolded over several years, I have seen the practice develop and language emerge for it as art therapists innovate and reflect on what they do with it and then share that with others. Conversations and research in the literature seem to move the work in community art therapy forward, with calls to continually define and redefine what art therapy is and does (Moon, 2000; Talwar, 2016). I have read the terms *social action art therapy* (Kaplan, 2007), *social art therapy* (Holingsbee, 2019), *community-based art therapy* (Ottemiller & Awais, 2016), *public practice art therapy* (Timm-Bottos, 2017), *festival art therapy* (Whitaker, 2021), and *museum-based art therapy* (Reyhani Dejkameh & Shipps, 2018), to name a few, and all seem to be types of art therapy that involve community practice. Language in the field is evolving as art therapists innovate practice.

Yet, in my own experience I have noticed that art therapists are not only averse to pinning down art therapy because it is adaptable in so many ways, but also, I think, out of fear that reducing it to a definition will spoil it. Art therapy is such a beautiful thing that no one wants to name it and claim it, for fear of losing it, but I do think that practitioners can name it and continue to stay present with it as it evolves and changes, continually redefining it as needed. An identified need exists to determine common therapeutic factors in art therapy (Robb, 2022) and clarify the theories of art therapy (Huss, 2015) so that art therapists can provide effective treatment. While providing verification for efficacy, with growth and evolution there is also a continued need to understand how art therapists aim to approach their work as they innovate. A few art therapists have developed concepts attending to efficacy in community art therapy practice.

Internal Studio

Kalmanowitz and Lloyd (1997, 2005) and Moon (2002) have distinguished that when working in the art therapy studio, the art therapist carries the structure of that studio internally, so that the studio is "portable" and adaptable to many different contexts. The art therapist in community contexts shares their portable studio with the participants. The studio in community can seemingly pop up anywhere and any time there are materials and people together. The participants' creative actions and interactions in community art therapy develop their own sense of an internal studio. The art therapist supports safe, healthy relationships with self, others, and the art, with opportunities for creativity, exploration, and authenticity (Nolan, 2019). The art made in studio is done in relationship to self, others, experience, environment, culture, and is an act of resilience. Resilience is being able to continue again and again after experiencing any internal and/or external struggle. Art becomes an act of resilience when a person has the inner capacity to devote to creation rather than survival.

Art Hives and Open Studios

Two art therapy specific examples of community art therapy in the literature are art hives and open studios. In the art hives described by Timm-Bottos and Chainey (2015) the hive operates out of the belief that everyone is an artist, who is welcomed and included; the approach celebrates the strengths and creativity of the individual and community, encourages self-directed creative actions through diverse art material options, learning, and skill sharing, promotes emerging leadership in all ages, shares resources, provides free access through gift economy, and continually sows seeds of social change.

The open studio process was first conceived by Allen (1983), even though there is a rich history that has evolved to help develop open studio language (Hogan, 2001; Kramer, 2000; Moon, 2015; Pittman, 2016; Wix, 2000).

> The main features of the open studio approach emphasize artistic creation and provide the venue and conditions for this process. The artmaking process is not directed or moderated by the facilitators, and the sessions, deliberately longer than clinical sessions, enable profound engagement and sufficient time for the creative process to evolve.
>
> (Finkel & Bat Or, 2020, p. 2)

The open studio approach is generally a social one and has been applied in many different contexts, both clinical and non-clinical (Moon, 2015). Because of its social nature, flexibility, and adaptability the open studio works well in community contexts.

Grounded Theory Methods

Theory is a framework that is used to view related concepts about a topic, and grounded theory is developed from systematically collected data (Charmaz, 2014). "The goal of grounded theory is to develop theories based on people's lived experiences rather than proving or disproving existing theories" (Brown, 2017, p. 33). I find that theory and practice work in tandem, and that theory must be supported by what is happening, in this case community practice in the field of art therapy. Presented here, the experience of art therapy practitioners working in communities around the world shaped this grounded theory of the definition and approaches of community art therapy. Art therapy practitioners were asked how they define community art therapy and how they work with communities. Each theoretical idea emerged in conversations with practicing community art therapy facilitators and all the common factors have been synthesized through my own knowledge and experiences as an art therapist, professor, and community practitioner to construct a beehive model of community art therapy.

Definitions of Community Art Therapy

Community Art Therapy Is Both an Approach and a Setting

When art therapist Luisa Mariño works in any art therapy environment, her intention is to use a community approach. She hopes to facilitate spaces that are safe, both physically and psychologically, and encourage participants to explore topics such as stigma in collectivist cultures, which can become barriers in therapeutic and/or group processes. Mariño said:

> I'm from Colombia and the arts in themselves have played a huge role in how people can communicate to cope with parts of our shared history and traumas. I've found it even more now that I practice, very relevant to make art not only individually but also as a community. And here [in the United States], which is something that I didn't think about before getting myself familiarized with the political and diverse cultural context, creating in community can foster a sense of belonging—both in the specific space where the group is taking place and within a larger community, where otherwise you perhaps wouldn't feel that you belong and feeling maybe like—the other [alienated].

She said that she aims to have people explore and adjust the internal narrative or stories they believe about themselves, for example from "I'm shameful" to "I'm brave." Mariño leverages the people and the experiences they share in the community to amplify the strengths of each person and the community as a whole. She aims to create spaces where people feel they belong.

Leara Glinzak created a giant loom on wheels in a garage. Her intention was to use weaving and the loom to build connections between the residents of Grand Rapids, Michigan beyond their own neighborhoods. She brought the loom to areas where people were gathered, bringing art therapy to the community. She timed where she took the loom so that people could participate. She invited people to contribute to the community tapestry with a color, word, or image. People became curious, participated, and even began to write messages to, and respond to, one another. Throughout this project and process Glinzak was thinking through the lens of community practice. Although her interactions with participants and the loom were individual, her intention was to create connection among people in her community.

Traditionally, a setting in art therapy is any place where someone receives art therapy services. The setting often refers to a place of treatment such as a school, hospital, inpatient or outpatient clinic, private practice, community, etc. Many hospitals in the United States, Canada, Australia, the UK, and other areas offer art therapy. One way to explore the idea of both/and regarding setting and approach is by looking at a typical clinical setting, such as a hospital, which offers medical art therapy and often uses clinical art therapy approaches with individual patients and groups. Yet, here in Milwaukee, I see that some hospitals also offer community art therapy studios and programs open to the general hospital community and the public. In this example, the setting is medical, but the approach uses the lens of community treatment.

In contrast, art therapists Karina Donald and Lesli Ann Belnavis-Elliot work in Grenada and Jamaica respectively. They noted that they do not use the term *community art therapy* with participants because in these collectivist societies, community is inherent. When they work with participants, they are always considering the community; it is the water they swim in and the air that they breathe. Community is the way they view their work, regardless of working with an individual or a group.

Many art therapists working in the community know about aspects of the psychological, social, cultural, historical, and sometimes spiritual contexts of the people they work with, the systems that influence their clients, and the effects of therapy on those systems and society. Art therapists in community acknowledge where their communities and the individuals in them hold power in effectuating personal and community change, and where they feel powerless. The perspectives of the community art therapy practitioner are wide; they consider the benefits of art therapy on not only the individual but also the group, and how those benefits interplay with the systems that they are embedded within and affected by.

Community Art Therapy Is Practiced in Context and Shaped by Culture

Community art therapy is practiced in the contexts of people's daily lives. The way that culture embeds the arts in the daily life of the community influences how people welcome, accept, or reject community art therapy. Culture is created by the history, actions, and interactions of the people within it; it is dynamic and ever-changing. The arts are used within cultures and communities differently, and art therapists apply that knowledge in how they engage people in art therapy. Gina Alfonso and Magis Creative Spaces provided art therapy services to a community in the Philippines that had experienced devastation from a typhoon. The art therapists realized that the community used dance as a ritual. Rather than bringing to the community art materials that they may never have used or seen before or will have access to afterwards, the therapists used dance in their therapeutic work there. As Gina Alfonso said, they wanted to make sure that they were "honoring [the community's] own cultural traditions and integrating that in the process of offering everybody psychosocial support." In this way, the materials that are used in practice have cultural relevance to the group. Kapitan et al. (2011) found that cross-cultural art therapy experiences must be sensitive to the local conditions and require adept and humble facilitation. Art therapists adapt to meet needs; this includes using art materials that are easily accessed in that location and whose use requires no specialized knowledge.

Many art therapy practitioners around the world are educated in places outside of those where they work. Some art therapists have been educated in places that hold individualism as a societal value yet practice in places that are collectivist, specifically those therapists who have been trained in the UK or the United States and practice in Asia, Central America, and parts of Africa. In some areas where art therapists are working, art therapy is not recognized as a formal profession through regulatory credentialing, such as Hong Kong and Vietnam, or is only just developing, such as in Latvia and Croatia. The conflicting experiences between how one has been educated and how they practice challenges art therapists to reflect on their training and assess the needs of the people they are working with, and to then adapt their practice accordingly. Julia Byrne noted that, "Any good therapeutic intervention needs to outlast the therapy itself." This is an acute reflection in any therapeutic context, but here applies to knowing how to develop art therapy experiences that are relevant to the people and the culture in a community. This includes understanding family dynamics, who holds power in the culture and how they hold it, typical social expectations, culturally approved modes of expressing thoughts and emotion, and accepted forms of creativity and artmaking. The self-reflexivity of the art therapy practitioner is crucial in order to be able to adapt art therapy learnings from one cultural context to another.

In places where art therapy is a developing field, an art therapist who employs self-reflexivity can hold awareness of that if they use more traditional art therapy approaches this could lead to colonizing that geographical area (Hocoy, 2007). "Art therapy—and the psychology it is based on—originated in the global North and West and has been exported to different parts of the world, unconsciously replicating colonial patterns of cultural domination" (Kapitan et al., 2011, p. 64).

Effective art therapy offered in any area is nuanced to be relevant to the local cultural practice of the arts; it needs to include an understanding of the political, health, and educational systems in place that impact the community and the resources of the area to sustain any further services; and should provide those who participate with needed additional resources.

Art therapists in Peru, Germany, the United States, among other places, are working with people who are refugees from oppressive forces such as war, and other political or environmental upheavals. Families are displaced, often into camps in harboring countries, and the art therapists adapt their methods to the cultures of the people coming in. Carolyn Krüger works in refugee camps in Germany, and she found that she needed to make relationships with the families to assess the best ways to help the children in the studio. Due to dislocation, the culture of the camps was changing and developing depending on the makeup of the groups present. She worked mostly in community groups but would set aside time to work with individual children if it helped them to participate in community art therapy.

Community Art Therapy Centers' Creative Practices for Individual and Collective Therapeutic and Transformational Benefits

One of the primary intentions of community art therapy is for individuals and the collective to experience therapeutic and transformational benefits from making art. Community art therapy and community arts have much in common; they both offer outlets for social creativity and action. However, they differ in that the primary objectives within community art therapy are that people experience both therapeutic *and* transformational processes and outcomes. In community arts contexts the therapeutic gains are secondary, and art indirectly supports and empowers the community. This appears specifically in terms of both the process of artmaking and the product of it. In art therapy, both the process and the product are valued and important (Thompson, 2009).

Working with a local community arts agency in Milwaukee, I experienced that when there was a public viewing of the artwork from a specific project organization, leaders wanted to make sure that the product was aesthetically pleasing, using the elements and principles of design in a cohesive and engaging way. The leaders placed a lot of aesthetic importance on the resultant art product to potentially gain more funding for future projects. The art product was valued over any sort of personal or community therapeutic engagement in the artmaking process and at times seemed to undermine the participatory goals of the program. I worked with one program that included child participants that had an adult artist-in-residence. The adult artist designed the work without input from the children or community, but with approval from the community arts agency, and then painted over the children's work to make it more "presentable." Now, not all community arts agencies are like this; many artists are trained in and uphold community principles, but there can be a tension when collaborating with community arts, and positive outcomes necessitate lots of discussion about not only what the community ideals are but also what art therapy is and how it plays a role.

Part of what takes place in dialog within community art therapy projects is this idea of intention and negotiating what is therapeutic. Some art therapists mentioned that they are very explicit in how they communicate that the program is therapeutic, while others mention that they focus less on this to engage more people without discouraging participants because of stigma or lack of awareness and understanding of art therapy.

Community Art Therapy Continues to Grow and Evolve

Art therapy continues to grow and evolve, as does community art therapy. Art therapists have identified that this happens in several ways. Art therapy develops as there is more awareness about what it is, as new practices are innovated. Art therapy evolves as more education and training programs are offered and it is recognized as a profession in more locations. Art therapists support the growth of the field when they build relationships with other art therapists, forming their own supportive and collaborative practitioner communities.

Community efforts have helped art therapists bring awareness to the field and educate the public. As larger-scale efforts have taken off in certain regions, art therapists notice that there is an interest, and participation, in what they do, often followed by media coverage. Art therapists have raised consciousness about the field by educating other practitioners in related fields. As they talk about their work and how art therapy is adaptable to meet needs in many different settings, other professionals have begun to refer their clients and people in their own communities.

Awareness spreads through new and fun ways that art therapy is happening, such as at festivals and in shopping malls. Art therapists describe many ways of innovating practice. Projects and programs have been held in many places as practitioners go to where people are in the community and bring art therapy with them. "Pop-up" art therapy studios have appeared in many likely and unlikely places, focusing on wellness and self-care, to create a one-time experience—places such as farmers' markets, sporting events, wellness fairs, music festivals, etc. Many unlikely collaborators have helped with this innovation. In one neighborhood in Hong Kong, Bianca Lee collaborated with beauty queens to reduce the mental health stigma of seeking help. Beauty queens are so well loved in Hong Kong that their participation helped to provide credibility. In another program Lee held in a shopping mall, snow was brought in as an art material. Snow in Hong Kong is rarely seen, let alone played in; the material was so novel that people were able to explore, have fun, and experience temporality.

In many areas of the world, the profession of art therapy is not recognized. Without awareness and recognition, there is also a lack of regulation. In some ways, implementing regulation is a barrier to work, blocking necessary innovation, but in other ways it protects the public and establishes baseline conditions for education and training. Art therapy is in varying stages of development worldwide and arises out of the different political experiences of each country. The way that art therapy is recognized and regulated, or not, depends on the health systems and infrastructure of those places.

Heartwarmingly, art therapists everywhere are building communities among themselves to support each other. As practitioners build their networks of professionals, they are working together to create coalitions of art therapists and, in areas such as North America, Europe, and Asia, even formal professional associations, and organizations. Many art therapists educated outside of the geographical area where they are working have described feeling shame as they have adapted their training to practice in their current cultures and contexts; they report feeling as though they are abandoning professional art therapy ideals because they weren't taught that there would be a need to adapt their learning. Creating a community of art therapists helps them to support one another and feel their own sense of interdependence and interconnectedness.

Community Art Therapy Approaches

Practitioners set up conditions for the community to experience the available therapeutic factors, using art materials and processes. As noted by Robb (2022), common therapeutic factors in group art therapy, which can extend to community groups, include expression, awareness, interpersonal engagement, and creativity. The following are the necessities that art therapy practitioners have identified as they work in and with communities.

Community Art Therapy Is Practiced Skillfully and Ethically

Art therapists work ethically in all contexts, and in community art therapy this is no different. However, those ethics may not be formally explicated in areas where art therapy is developing, and as art therapy grows, it is important that ethics emerge with practice and are defined by responses within the community. Art therapists working in communities approach their work with cultural humility and sensitivity. They navigate personal disclosure, boundaries, and multiple roles carefully, often with guidance from other more experienced practitioners, and from the community itself. Art therapists offer art materials that are familiar to participants and easily accessed once the program or project is complete, or the participants bring materials. The ethics and unique skills of the practitioners in community art therapy are so important that they are covered in depth in Chapter 5.

Community Art Therapy Is Inclusive, Accessible, and Provides People with a Place and Sense of Belonging

Inclusive

Creating safe, inclusive spaces requires not only that everybody is accepted into the community space but also that they know that they are invited. Facilitators understand their responsibility to be aware of their own identities, power, and privileges in relation to the people in their community as well as the historical, social, and cultural contexts of the geographical area.

In community spaces of inclusion, representation matters, along with a careful questioning of who is invited into the space and who is facilitating in it. Do the identities of the facilitators reflect the identities of the group members? If not, then why not? And if not, how does the facilitator communicate that they are an ally, ready to be in authentic relationship, without being performative?

Colombian art therapist, Ana García has hosted many art hives for Spanish speakers; she supports inclusion and belonging through language. Inclusive practices consider the dominant language spoken by the community and then offer opportunities to engage by providing facilitators who speak the language or by bringing in interpreters. This is a common occurrence in refugee camps or other mixed cultural spaces, where it is less likely that art therapists will represent the identities of the participants.

Accessible

Community art therapy programs and projects can be offered where the community is located, rather than expecting the community to come to art therapy. I founded an art therapy organization that offers both community and clinical art therapy opportunities—Bloom Art and Integrated Therapies, Inc, in Milwaukee, Wisconsin. During my dissertation research, Bloom offered a studio at a daytime shelter for those experiencing homelessness and one at the organization's own premises. Comparing the two community art therapy studios, I saw a marked difference in the time it took to build a regular attendance at the studio in Bloom—almost two years; but when the art therapists went to the daytime shelter for those experiencing homelessness, the community developed much more quickly, and within weeks there was regular attendance. Going to the community, and to the places where the community lives, makes it easier for people to access services, especially considering any barriers such as limited transport or available time for travel. Focusing on how to support people's ability to participate may impact their willingness to attend; in the daytime shelter for people experiencing homelessness, I saw that they were more likely to come to art therapy because they felt respected in being offered the opportunity in a familiar place. Going out to where participants already are helps them to feel that they are viewed as important and valued, and so they attend more readily.

Community experiences can be a conduit for a person entering clinical treatment. Clinical treatment is not always needed, nor is it always the therapeutic goal, but sometimes it is necessary. Having a positive experience in the community, where individuals feel accepted, included, while a sense of belonging is fostered, can help transition participants to other art therapy or mental health services. For some, community art therapy is also a way *out* of treatment. People discharged from inpatient facilities and into the community can engage in community art therapy projects that provide a bridge between their inpatient experiences and community life.

Community art therapy presents a liminal space that can trigger an interest or trust in moving into a different and more personal experience. In my experience, the community art therapy studios we offer at Bloom have been a safe way for people to reenter the community after a hospitalization or several individual sessions. The transitional opportunity that community art therapy offers expands possibilities of treatment and meets clients where they are in their healing and transformation.

Countries the world over are seeking ways to improve access to care. Mental health issues occur worldwide and affect 25% of the population (Coêlho et al., 2021). Providing more opportunities to engage in treatment is one way of increasing access. As art therapy continues to develop, hopefully so too will the availability of training. The more art therapists there are available, the more services there will be, increasing societal awareness of art therapy and its capacities for transformation. "When a whole community embraces the idea of art as a healing technology and applies it to its own particular needs, a thousand permutations become possible" (Kapitan, 2008, p. 2). As art therapists and communities widen their notions of how, when, where, and by whom treatment can be offered, community practices will play a major role in accessibility of health care services. Community endeavors increase the number of people who can engage in art therapy, providing a more cost-effective way of providing services. From a liberatory and critical standpoint, this establishes increased opportunity to engage in art therapy and increases accessibility to services offered, not just for those with means but also for those who have been excluded, historically.

Accessibility also applies to art materials and processes, which appropriately come from within the culture and context of the geographical location of the program. However, in general, accessibility can refer to ensuring that all materials and processes are suitable for the age, physical, and cognitive abilities of the people in the community. Community participants can bring in their own materials for use. We had a group at Bloom that wanted to use clay, but we did not have any clay available to us. The art therapists consulted with the group about what types of clay they could get, and the group brought their own. Often, Bloom and the agencies we work with receive donated materials. Organizations can put out a call for specific donations, or see what materials happen to come in. Once, Bloom got a large donation of material samples from a local upholstery business; it was exciting to see what people made from the fabric.

Community art therapy studios offer directive and non-directive artmaking opportunities. Directive means that there is a structured process or product-making that the participants will engage in. For example, the participants explore materials or themes based on the directions of the facilitator. Non-directive means that there is no structure or process to follow, and several material options are provided and the choice of what to do or make is up to the participants. Some studios offer both processes at the same time. In many programs, and specifically the daytime shelter studio at Bloom, art therapists use a combination of approaches to ensure accessibility. Some people can explore on their own and others need a place, and a structure, from which to start.

Belonging

A person experiences a sense of belonging when they feel they are a part of something, experiencing a real connection with others, while being able to maintain their authenticity, power, and freedom (Brown, 2017). Fortune et al. (2021) researched belonging in older adults who participate in art hives that promote well-being by addressing isolation. The older adults who felt a sense of belonging in the art hives described that belonging requires nonjudgmental social spaces that they can attend for more reasons than artmaking alone, and that they were there to create a shared space with others. Although the research findings from art hives specifically attune to older adults, the learning may also be extended to effects found in non-aged participants who also attend the art hives. Contributing to art therapy as spaces of belonging, art therapists understand that people seek out places and activities where they feel they belong, where they are welcomed and accepted.

In one example, art therapist Elissa Arbeitman holds a community group for women that uses a painting process. She contends that, "women need a place to be held in their wholeness." One way that she facilitates with belonging in mind is by establishing the norm that the women will show up however they are feeling, and she encourages communication within the group to show that members accept each other.

However, while "being social may be imperative, … it is not always easy" (Dissanayake, 2000, p. 57). Most community art therapists described the incredible importance of facilitating art therapy spaces of belonging so that people feel as if they fit with and are accepted by others. Moon and Shuman (2013) describe that belonging requires *radical* acceptance. Rather than privilege neurotypical behavior, sometimes a harm-reduction mindset is adopted in the culture of the community. This mindset can challenge notions of safety as opposed to feelings of discomfort. In one type of situation Moon shared, if someone presents high or drunk, but they are not physically or emotionally hurting anyone, then the group continues to welcome them in. The art therapist facilitates this with the group encouraging discussion among the members to build and strengthen connection.

Moon holds the safety of the space but may challenge the social norms associated with safety through discussion. However, this may not be acceptable in all community situations.

I agree that creating spaces of belonging may seem like a simple concept, but it is actually very complex. People are accepted in the community as they are, without a belief that they must fit into strict inclusion criteria; however, community art therapy spaces are created within the context of the culture, both to follow and carefully question the norms of that culture to create social change.

Community Art Therapy Addresses Social Issues and Inequities

Community art therapy practitioners strive to provide opportunities to address social issues in the social realm. Offering social solutions to social problems powerfully advocates for community, cultural, and systemic change (Kaplan, 2007; Hocoy, 2007; Talwar, 2019). Social issues include social isolation; relational trauma, collective trauma, transgenerational trauma, and environmental trauma; systemic oppression; violence based on race, religion, sexuality, gender, and disability; political conflict, upheaval, and violence; economic hardship; and lack of basic needs, such as food, shelter, or adequate medical care. Community art therapy endeavors to address social issues among those who may be experiencing similar issues by inviting opportunities to collectively dream, express, and plan how they might be able to creatively resolve those issues, seek justice, or simply provide solidarity and validation for each other.

All over the world, stigma regarding mental illness and treatment exists. Community art therapy offers a counter experience to stigma. Community efforts focused on wellness and creativity are a "softer entry" into therapy, said Rozanne Myburgh. She also noted that, for some, making art with others, rather than attending an individual session focused on addressing personal or societal problems, is far less scary. Additionally, community art therapy opportunities help to break down prejudices and stereotypes when they bring diverse people together in one place focused on creativity and wellness. People can engage with others who are different and then decenter their own experience, which opens them up to changing their perspective while challenging their assumptions and biases.

In the Philippines, creative therapeutic community programs amplified the rich cultural traditions of typically underrepresented indigenous groups by engaging with the mainstream culture through performance of traditional dance rituals. To counter the indigenous group's lack of feeling accepted by mainstream/dominant culture, they were able to share information about the culture's roots and identity with the dominant group within the culture, reversing the notion of the "haves" and the "have nots." The indigenous groups became the "haves" when members of the mainstream culture acknowledged the knowledge and power the indigenous group holds in being keepers of their rich history.

In Croatia, young and elderly art therapy participants were asked what they would like to build together. In Latvia, communities were asked to write letters to a future Latvia. Many art therapists work with communities in a future-oriented way, and Kalmanowitz and Lloyd (2005) have described that in the art therapy studio, "the present, past and future can find context" (p. 117). By dreaming of a future, the community acknowledges what has happened in the past and looks to future solutions holding onto hope. Community art therapy offers hopefulness, which seems to be a necessity in places that have experienced a collapse of government, war, and social unrest.

Health care systems and structures in many places, including any type of mental health therapy, are developing, specifically in Eastern Europe, areas of Africa, Asia, and Central America. In some of those areas, community art therapy has developed before individual treatment or as an alternative to it because of lack of access to health care and basic resources. "Social justice in ... art therapy ... translates into understanding how clients are positioned in society and if they have equal and fair access to resources and benefits" (Talwar, 2019, p. 11.) Community art therapy developed in those areas because of a significant need for mental health services and advocacy for social change.

Community Art Therapy Expands Practice Beyond Intrapsychic Frameworks and the Medical Model of Care

In Jamaica, a group of kids ran out of their school building, and Lesli Ann Belnavis-Elliot ran after them. She had to think fast about what to do next. In Jamaica, there is a phrase, "Tun yuh han mek fashion," meaning you use whatever you can, and you make it work. She began to sing and gather the children up in a circle. With the children looking at her incredulously, but with no other thought on how to proceed, she started a call and response. She was there as an art therapist to address a death by shooting of one of the children in the class. She began to chant, "When the gunshot fire, them ..." And the children would respond with their answer, slowly beginning to sing along. The game of call and response gained their trust and cooperation, and the content of the call and response helped them begin to process what had happened. Belnavis-Elliot uses art to gain trust and build relationship, communicate, and uses a sensory experience; all of these enhance therapeutic value.

In community art therapy the work is oriented toward prevention, attending to wellness, restoration, resilience, and connecting people to hope. In Germany, Carolyn Krüger was working in a refugee camp with children and described how unethical it would have been for her to have focused on an exploration of the internal material of the participants while they were so vulnerable. Although art therapy with individuals can be focused on intrapsychic exploration, in social settings, when working with internal material wouldn't be appropriate, the method shifts to include psychosocial approaches. Thus, practicing ethically and in a community-centered way focuses on strengths and resilience.

Psychodynamic frameworks typically rely on bringing unconscious material to the level of consciousness to resolve internal conflicts. Many training programs teach this framework and, historically, in Western contexts, it has been an idealized form of treatment in art therapy (Robb, 2022). Community art therapy expands what art therapy is and how it is practiced, reaching beyond intrapsychic treatment. In community art therapy the work is relational-focused, strengths-based, integrated, and aligned with Bucciarelli's (2016) transdisciplinary conceptualization.

> Art therapy is an integrated combination of art techniques and processes, psychological theories, educational models, sociocultural constructs, and biological understandings. … requiring integration of all these knowledge areas; art therapy cannot be practiced by excluding any one area. As such, art therapists are encouraged to work comprehensively and inclusively, but also flexibly.
>
> (p. 152)

Following a medical model, to be included in a therapy group in a hospital and an outpatient setting requires a diagnosis. Most community art therapy groups do not have this requirement, even though some people who participate may have a diagnosis. Community art therapy practitioners think about the social, cultural, and historical contexts of the participants, their relationships, and individual and collective behavior, thoughts, emotions, sensations, and experiences. Participants in many community art therapy programs, such as in Croatia, Serbia, Philippines, Colombia, and other places, have been affected by, and displaced due to, environmental trauma, war, or political harm; no diagnosis could be given for such an experience. "Dominant culture frameworks for normality and psychopathology such as the *DSM* [*Diagnostic and Statistical Manual of Mental Disorders*, used in the United States] frequently mask the relationship between the symptoms that are expressed by individuals and societal imbalances"; this then "situates the problem within the individual rather than the within the broader collective context" (Hocoy, 2007, pp. 25–26). Communities in art therapy "can focus on relationships, connection, and repair rather than symptom reduction" (Robb, 2022, p. 6). Community art therapy practice expands and evolves the medical model to include social models that provide a wholistic approach to growth, wellness, therapy, and transformation.

Community art therapy has certainly expanded practice at Lefika la Phodiso in South Africa. "What goes on back there?" the teen community art therapy participants often ask the creative therapists about the private sessions that have started at the center. Rozanne Myburgh noted that the positive experiences in the community have led many youths to be curious about individual sessions. Until recently, to provide access, the programs offered were only community-based, but there has been an increasing need to address individual concerns in private sessions.

Community Art Therapy Encourages Interdependent and Egalitarian Relationships

Everyone is conceived through relational contact, then gestates in the womb, and at birth relies on others for feeding and care; people need connection with others to thrive. Community art therapy encourages interdependent relationships and promotes interconnectedness through shared accountability, purpose, resources, expression, such as storytelling and creativity while collaborating with community leaders, other disciplines, and other organizations.

Art therapists understand and share the values of the community they are working within. Community art therapy is participatory and encourages dialogue and negotiation in terms of shared decision-making; in this way, the power within the community is shared. María Cristina Ruiz Echeverry practices in Colombia and isn't interested in working in non-collective art therapy endeavors that don't share power. She works with children in community, sharing her skills in puppetry. However, art therapists must understand the limits of their shared power; this concept is covered in more depth in Chapter 4.

Participants in community art therapy include the art therapy provider, other facilitators, community leaders, and anyone else who is engaged in the project. Community leaders are often called upon to participate and collaborate as an important resource. Sarah Baker in Pittsburgh, PA, interviewed the community to develop a plan for a mural. She met with community members and leaders to hear the voices of all the community stakeholders, then brought what she had learned back to the teens she works with at the drop-in community center, and together they created a concept drawing of the mural.

Programs are integrated with other therapeutic arts, providing opportunities to connect to multiple modes of expression, creativity, advocacy, and healing as well as local resources. Oihika Chakrabarti, an art therapist, worked through her non-profit, Manahkshetra Foundation (art for social change), with the Kala Ghoda Festival in 2005 in Mumbai—the largest arts festival in India—to create a photographic installation outside the Jehangir Art gallery and Prince of Wales Museum that developed a citizens' initiative to bring art out of museums and gallery spaces to make it relevant to people from all walks of life. The project was based on the premise that there is a latent artist in everyone that should be celebrated, and solicited photographs from the public that captured the spirit of the city. Students of the J.J. College of Art participated in work with street children in various localities and were given cameras to photograph their neighborhoods. All submitted photographs were included in the installation, and they tied in to a Bollywood theme, which is pervasive in Mumbai, and included street kitsch and excerpts from Indian authors celebrating the city through their writings, poetry, and films as part of the festival. That year, the arts festival in the city had the largest footfall on record. The following year the installation was converted to a film format and screened at the Prince of Wales Museum during the Kala Ghoda Arts festival, with plans to convert it to a coffee-table book titled *Aamchi Mumbai* (Our Mumbai) People's Album. These connections are empowering and carry projects or programs forward as social capital is gained through networking with as many local resources as possible (Allen, 2007). Joining with collaborators and integrating with local resources contributes to the sustainability of healthy individuals and communities even after projects or programs end and the potential power of the arts gets redefined in an entirely new way.

In art therapy, people validate one another and experience being seen, heard, and understood. Participants can feel empowered by sharing their expertise with others and being open to learning new skills and ideas from their peers; "each one teach one" (Timm-Bottos & Chainey, 2015). Community art therapy seeks to build interconnectedness through offering occasions for reciprocal learning and sharing of skills, stories, and art.

People can find resonance with one another in sharing their images and their similar experiences. Luisa Mariño offered that often in her groups, participants would call out someone's bravery by asking, "Did you hear yourself say that?" Participants can inadvertently become mirrors for one another's achievements, progress, and resilience; for example, when acknowledging others' strengths and courage. Participants sometimes may not embrace themselves until they have witnessed someone else's healing.

Community art therapy can be a space of refuge and/or a bridge to the larger community. Community art therapy studios offer small spaces of refuge within larger communities through access, inclusion, and belonging (Moon & Shuman, 2013). Studio members of Bloom's community art therapy studio in the daytime shelter for people experiencing homelessness called it "a refuge within a refuge." And, when the products and experiences of community art therapy are safely shared with the wider community—for example, through exhibiting artwork—the opportunity is offered to further connection, reduce stigma, and expand who is included in community.

bell hooks (2003) noted that societies are socialized to believe that domination and hierarchy are necessary. "In actuality, to intervene in dominator culture, to live consciously, we must be willing to share with anyone knowledge about how to make the transition from a dominator model to a partnership model" (hooks, 2003, p. 76). Unlike in the medical model, which holds the practitioner up as an expert, connection through non-hierarchical relationships values all participants as experts and equals, sharing their various talents and knowledge with each other and creating relationships that provide mutual support. Thahmina Begum worked with Bangladeshi adults in the UK to address racism. She sees the importance of meeting people where they are at, helping the trauma that happens in the community to be healed in the community. Healing is supported by the connections of each person present, without regard to hierarchy. When *everyone* makes art together to address a social concern and common experience, then, "Art can be the unspeakable thing that connects us all." Therapeutic community activities offer an alternative to the mainstream mental health treatment patient/provider hierarchy through establishing and encouraging a culture of community care that invites people to care for and support one another.

Training Non–Art Therapists Furthers Interdependence and Interconnection on a Wider Scale

In many parts of the world, art therapy as a field is growing and developing, but in these places there is a lack of opportunity and access to formal art therapy training. Art therapists have trained non–art therapists to be practitioners in these places. Kapitan et al. (2011) have utilized what they call the "multiplier effect," training community leaders to use art therapy, who then go back to their local areas to share what they have learned.

Another way to look at this is known as task shifting/sharing. "Task shifting is a process of delegation whereby tasks are moved, where appropriate, to less specialized health workers" (Keshri & Garg, 2021, p. 253). Task sharing is the collaborative effort, between providers with different levels of training, to share tasks (Orkin et. al., 2021). Task shifting and sharing has developed out of the need for more efficient health resources. In community art therapy it refers to collaboration between art therapy professionals and other professionals who may be skilled in areas such as medicine, psychology, nursing, or education who can be trained in art therapy skills that may be of use in a community context and then supervised by art therapists to complete the work. This is explored further in Chapter 5; here it is presented as an example of interdependence in action. Task shifting and sharing is a scaled version of *each one–teach one*, often employed in many art hives (Timm-Bottos & Chainey, 2015), and can have an impact on accessibility, who is included in the community, and societal change. (More information about training non–art therapists is included in Chapter 5.)

Community Art Therapy Is Embodied and Supports Nervous System Regulation

In US and UK contexts, a disconnect often exists between the human brain and the human body. A common observation is that artmaking involves all parts of the body and can help regulate the nervous system. A regulated nervous system supports overall health (Kain & Terrell, 2018). Sally Goldstraw said she often encourages community members to, "Follow your hands to get out of your brain space." She sees the benefit of helping to quiet the executive functions of the brain to open a "sensory doorway." The doorway from the brain to the body facilitates access to creativity and healing.

Much research in the last 20 years in psychology and adjacent fields, such as art therapy, has focused on understanding the brain and how brain functions impact growth and healing. Alongside understanding the structures and functions of the brain has been explicating art therapy as an embodied practice, and how emotions and the nervous system are regulated. In my experience, if a person feels anxious, an art therapist is very naturally going to want to do two things: 1) help the client to eliminate or decrease the anxiety that they are feeling; or 2) help them increase their capacity to tolerate that feeling or emotion. Anxiety and any emotion that causes someone to feel activated in their body can get stuck in an unsettled state, conversely any emotion that causes settling, such as sadness, can get also cause one to get stuck in a deactivated state, such as depression. When someone gets caught in activated or deactivated state this can result in dysregulation (Levine, 2010). From a trauma perspective, the goal would be to increase the window of tolerance between high levels of activation and low levels of settling, and then regulate the nervous system (Ogden & Minton, 2000). Regulating the nervous system allows a free flow between the appropriate activation and rest of the nervous system.

Making marks on paper using rhythm and repetition is a kinesthetic action, which supports tapping into the wisdom of the body (Hinz, 2019). Often using all five senses in artmaking, or offering multisensory experiences, promotes the ability to self-soothe and supports regulation. This is also true of other creative expressions that utilize kinesthetic and sensory channels; for example, dance is used in many collective cultural rituals. In the Philippines, Gina Alfonso saw that, having experienced a tsunami, the community danced together every Saturday evening as a way of celebrating all they had that remained, comforting themselves, and collectively resetting their nervous systems. Lesli Ann Belnavis-Elliot described using rhythm through call and response to engage the school community and encourage co-regulation. She also observed that the children would make a call-and-response and then run to the fence and back and then start the call-and-response again. Very naturally, they were titrating their own exposure to processing trauma. They all chanted, "When the gunshot fire, them …"; one child would respond with "hide under the bed," addressing the trauma; and then they would all run to the fence and back in the schoolyard to discharge the activation before coming back to face the trauma again.

Co-regulation, or regulating with others, is something that people are wired to do. "[O]ur brain and nervous system are not isolated, but interconnected and social. At our core, we are social beings who regulate through connection with others" (Heller, 2019, p. 6). Coherence reflects a homeostatic state in which the body is optimally self-regulating and overall stable (Somatic Experiencing Training Manual, 2022, p. 4). Research suggests that, in community, people can have a positive impact on each other's regulation and state of coherence (Edward, 2019; Morris, 2010). When people are coherent and self-regulated and hold the intention to impact others in the community positively, the level of coherence in other people's systems is affected.

Timm-Bottos (2006) shared that collective artmaking is a resource for creating resilience and experiencing joy, through establishing opportunities for people to play with materials during community experiences; interviews with art therapists practicing community art therapy confirm this. Linh Guyen works in Vietnam with people who are experiencing homelessness and guides art activities that invite play and curiosity. Encouraging opportunities for laughter and making creative mistakes taps into sharing joy with each other and is a resource for creating resilience—resilience being a way to bounce back time and again after experiencing trauma and setbacks. Carolyn Krüger, an art therapist who works with child refugees in Germany noticed that the children seemed to "hunger for the art materials because of the deprivation" they were experiencing. She invited play and fostered opportunities to use the art materials for regulation in the studio. As communities come to rely on interconnection and co-regulation through shared creative expression and artmaking, they can positively influence each other's nervous systems and, potentially, their overall health.

A Beehive Model of Community Art Therapy

Community art therapy is like a beehive and the work of bees. Beehives are created by colonies of bees and each bee has a place in the hive ("Perfect Bee," 2022). Bees fulfill one of three roles in the colony—as a worker bee, a drone, or as the queen—and no role is more important than another. The queen bee with the drones, who are male, is responsible for the continued survival of the hive through procreation. The worker bees are female and work together to extract nectar, heat, cool, and guard the entrance to the hive, and build the hexagonal cells where nectar, honey, pollen, and larvae are stored. The process of storing pollen and making honey and wax, requires the actual comingling of fluids and enzymes between the worker bees. When the bees build more cells, this naturally expands the structure of the hive. Each of the combs is not more important than the other but are related and interconnected to further show how power is shared in the bee community. All the bees in the colony are socially minded and dependent on one another to ensure the colony thrives. Each bee is a vital contributor to the environment because they pollinate important foods that humans need for survival.

I conceptualized the beehive model of art therapy from the tenets of grounded theory to provide visual support and enhance understanding of how art therapists define and approach their community work (see Figure 2.1). The model shows that the structure of the hive is made up in the same way that community art therapy is defined; it is both an approach and a setting, shaped by culture, centers creative transformation for individuals and the collective, and continues to grow and evolve. The inner honeycombs of the hive offer objectives for art therapists when working in community practice.[1]

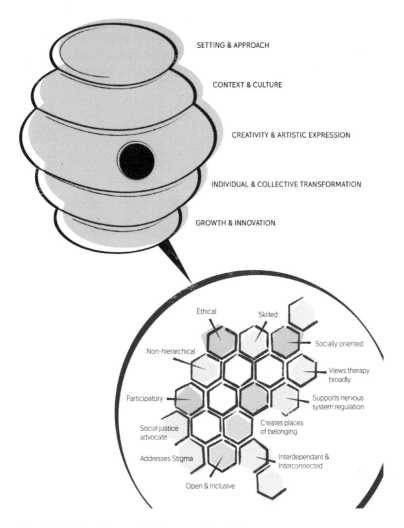

SETTING & APPROACH

CONTEXT & CULTURE

CREATIVITY & ARTISTIC EXPRESSION

INDIVIDUAL & COLLECTIVE TRANSFORMATION

GROWTH & INNOVATION

Ethical

Skilled

Non-hierarchical

Socially oriented

Views therapy broadly

Participatory

Supports nervous system regulation

Social justice advocate

Creates places of belonging

Addresses Stigma

Interdependant & Interconnected

Open & Inclusive

Figure 2.1 A beehive model of community art therapy

Conclusion

This chapter presents the definition and goals of community art therapy that have emerged in conversations with art therapists practicing in community around the world. The beehive model of community art therapy provides a visual representation of what community art therapy is and depicts the practice aims held in the honeycombs. Practiced together, the definition and aims presented here create a foundation where art therapists in community contexts can ground their practice and relate to each other with common language and goals. As this happens, art therapists working in community become a network; and that network creates shared power. Foucalt (1994) conceptualized power in this way; as people (the nodes) work together (circuits), they both experience and wield power. Art therapists with communities can wield power together for good and for healing.

Note

1 The research findings included in this chapter have also been submitted for publication in a scholarly journal. Some of what you are reading here may be published elsewhere.

References

Allen, P. (1983). Group art therapy in short-term hospital settings. *American Journal of Art Therapy*, *22*(3), 93–97.

Allen, P. (2007). Wielding the shield: The art therapist as conscious witness in the realm of social action. In F. Kaplan (Ed.), *Art therapy and social action* (pp. 72–85). Jessica Kingsley.

Brown, B. (2017). *Braving the wilderness: The quest for true belonging and the courage to stand alone*. Random House.

Bucciarelli, A. (2016). Art therapy: A transdisciplinary approach. *Art Therapy*, *33*(3), 151–155. https://doi.org/10.1080/07421656.2016.1199246

Charmaz, K. (2014). *Constructing grounded theory* (2nd ed.). Sage.

Coêlho, B., Santana, G., Viana, M., Wang, Y., & Andrade, L. (2021). "I don't need any treatment" – Barriers to mental health treatment in the general population of a megacity. *Brazilian Journal of Psychiatry*, *43*(6), 590–598. https://doi.org/10.1590/1516-4446-2020-1448

Dissanayake, E. (2000). *Art and intimacy*. University of Washington Press.

Edwards, S. D. (2019). The HeartMath coherence model: Implications and challenges for artificial intelligence and robotics. *AI and Society*, *34*(4), 899–905. https://doi.org/10.1007/s00146-018-0834-8

Finkel, D., & Bat Or, M. (2020). The open studio approach to art therapy: A systematic scoping review. *Frontiers in Psychology*, *11*, 568042. https://doi.org/10.3389/fpsyg.2020.568042

Fortune, D., Aubin, G., Timm-Bottos, J., & Hebblethwait, S. (2021). The art hive as a 'frame of belonging' for older adults. *Leisure/Loisir*, *45*(3), 459–480. https://doi.org/10.1080/14927713.2021.1886867

Foucault, M. (1994). *Dits et Écrits: 1954–1988*. Gallimard.

Heller, D. P. (2019). *The power of attachment: How to create deep lasting intimate relationships*. Sounds True.

Hinz, L. (2019). *Expressive therapies continuum: A framework for using art in therapy* (2nd ed.). Routledge.

Hocoy, D. (2007). Art therapy as a tool for social change: A conceptual model. In F. Kaplan (Ed.), *Art therapy and social action* (pp. 21–39). Jessica Kingsley.

Hogan, S. (2001). *Healing arts: The history of art therapy*. Jessica Kingsley.

Hollingsbee, E. (2019). 'Tomorrow we make it better': An art therapist's reflection on a community mural in a refugee camp in Greece. *International Journal of Art Therapy*, *24*(4), 158–168. https://doi.org/10.1080/17454832.2019.1666155

hooks, b (2003). *Teaching community: A pedagogy of hope*. Routledge.

Huss, E. (2015). *A theory-based approach to art therapy*. Routledge.

Inside and Out of the Beehive. (2022, December). *Perfect Bee*. Retrieved December 27, 2022, from https://www.perfectbee.com/learn-about-bees/the-life-of-bees/inside-and -out-of-the-beehive

Kain, K., & Terrell, S. (2018). *Nurturing resilience: Helping clients move forward from developmental trauma*. North Atlantic Books.

Kalmanowitz, D., & Lloyd, B. (1997). *The portable studio: Art therapy and political conflict: Initiatives in the former Yugoslavia and KwaZulu-Natal, South Africa*. Health Education Authority.

Kalmanowitz, D., & Lloyd, B. (2005). *Inside the portable studio in Art therapy and political violence: With art, without illusion* (D. Kalmanowitz & B. Lloyd, eds.). Routledge.

Kapitan, L. (2008). "Not art therapy": Revisiting the therapeutic studio in the narrative of the profession. *Art Therapy*, *25*(1), 2–3. https://doi.org/ 10.1080/07421656.2008.10129349

Kapitan, L., Litell, M., & Torres, A. (2011). Creative art therapy in a community's participatory research and social transformation. *Art Therapy*, *28*(2), 64–73. https:// doi.org/10.1080/07421656.2011.578238

Kaplan, F. (2007). Introduction. In F. Kaplan (Ed.), *Art therapy and social action* (pp. 11–17). Jessica Kingsley.

Keshri, V., & Garg, B. (2021). Operational barriers in providing comprehensive emergency obstetric care by task shifting of medical officers in selected states of India. *Indian Journal of Community Medicine*, *46*(2), 252–257.

Kramer, E. (2000). *Art as therapy*. Kingsley Publishers.

Moon, C. (2000). Art therapy, profession or idea? A feminist aesthetic perspective. *Art Therapy*, *17*(1), 7–10. https://doi.org/10.1080/07421656.2000.10129437

Moon, C. (2002). *Studio art therapy*. Jessica Kingsley Press.

Moon, C. (2015). Open studio approach to art therapy. In D. Gussak & M. Rosal (Eds.), *The Wiley handbook of art therapy*. (pp. 112–121). Wiley.

Moon, C., & Shuman, V. (2013). The community art studio: Creating a space of solidarity and inclusion. In P. Howie, S. Prasad, & J. Kristel (Eds.), *Using art therapy with diverse populations: Crossing cultures and abilities* (pp. 297–307). Jessica Kingsley.

Morris, S. (2010). Achieving collective coherence: Group effects on heart rate variability coherence and heart rhythm synchronization. *Alternative Therapies in Health and Medicine*, *16*(4), 62–72. http://tir-training.de/wp-content/uploads/2015/09/HeartMath _achieving-collective-coherence.pdf

Nolan, E. (2019). Opening art therapy thresholds: Mechanisms that influence change in the community art therapy studio. *Art Therapy*, *36*(2), 77–85. https://doi.org/10.1080 /07421656.2019.1618177

Levine, P. (2010). *In an unspoken voice: How the body releases trauma and restores goodness*. North Atlantic Books.

Ogden, P., & Minton, K. (2000). Sensory motor psychotherapy: One method for processing trauma. *Traumatology, 3*(3), 149–173.

Orkin, A., Rao, S., Venugopal, J., Kithulegoda, N., Wegier, P., Ritchie, S., VanderBurgh, D., Martiniuk, A., Salamanca-Buentello, F., & Upshur, R. (2021). Conceptual framework for task shifting and task sharing: An international Delphi study. *Human Resources for Health, 19*(61), 1–8. https://doi.org/10.1186/s12960-021-00605-z

Ottemiller, D., & Awais, Y. (2016). A model for art therapists in community-based practice. *Art Therapy, 33*(3), 144–150. https://doi.org/10.1080/07421656.2016.1199245

Pitman, A. (2016). Art as healing review. *BJPsychological Bulletin, 40*(1), 54. https://doi.org/ 10.1192/pb.bp.114.049544

Potash, J., Mann, S., Martinez, J., Roach, A., & Wallace, N. (2016). Spectrum of art therapy practice: Systematic literature review of *art therapy*, 1983–2014. *Art Therapy, 33*(3), 119–127. https://doi.org/10.1080/07421656.2016.1199242

Reyhani Dejkameh, M., & Shipps, R. (2018). From please touch to artaccess: The expansion of a museum-based art therapy program. *Art Therapy, 35*(4), 211–217. https://doi.org/10.1080/07421656.2018.1540821

Robb, M. (2022). *Group art therapy: Practice and research.* Routledge.

Somatic Experiencing Training Manual. (2022). *Advanced 1.* Somatic Experiencing International.

Talwar, S. (2016). Is there a need to redefine art therapy? *Art Therapy, 33*(3), 116–118. https://doi.org/10.1080/07421656.2016.1202001

Talwar, S. (2019). Beyond multiculturalism and cultural competence: A social justice vision in art therapy. In S. Talwar (Ed.), *Art therapy for social justice* (pp. 3–16). Routledge.

Thompson, G. (2009). Artistic sensibility in the studio and gallery model: Revisiting process and product. *Art Therapy, 26*(4), 159–166. https://doi.org/10.1080/07421656.2009.10129609

Timm-Bottos, J. (2006). Constructing creative community: Reviving health and justice through community arts. *Canadian Art Therapy Association Journal, 19*(2), 12–26. https://doi.org/10.1080/08322473.2006.11432285

Timm-Bottos, J. (2017). Public practice art therapy: Enabling spaces across North America (La pratique publique de l'art-thérapie: des espaces habilitants partout en Amérique du Nord). *Canadian Art Therapy Association Journal, 30*(2), 94–99. https://doi.org/10.1080/08322473.2017.1385215

Timm-Bottos, J., & Chainey, R. (2015). Art hives: How-to-guide. http://www.arthives.org/blog/art-hives-how- guide-le-guide-pratique-des-ruches-dart

Vick, M. (1996). The dimensions of service: An elemental model for the application of art therapy. *Art Therapy, 13*(2), 96–101. https://doi.org/10.1080/07421656.1996.10759202

Whitaker, P. (2021). Full on—Festival art therapy. *European Journal of Psychotherapy and Counselling.* https://doi.org/10.1080/13642537.2021.1961835

Wix, L. (2000). Looking for what's lost: The artistic roots of art therapy: Mary Huntoon. *Art Therapy, 17*(3), 168–176. https://doi.org/10.1080/07421656.2000.10129699

Chapter 3

Community Art Therapy Practice Reflections

*Emily Goldstein Nolan, Rochele Royster,
Lauren Leone, Ling Cheun Bianca Lee,
Angela Lyonsmith, Melissa Raman Molitor,
Louvenia Jackson, Gretchen M. Miller, Alison Tunis,
Pat B. Allen, Abbe Miller, Andrea Inés Velázquez Dorgan,
Chelsea O'Neil, Owen Karcher, Jennifer DeLucia,
Thahmina Begum, Lynn Kapitan, Laura Swift and
Dani Moss*

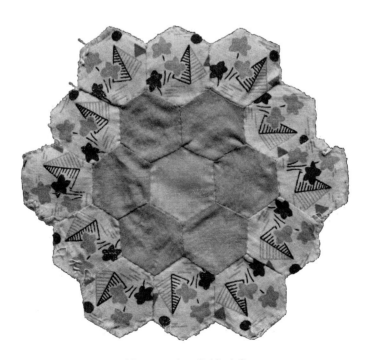

Honeycomb quilt block 3

DOI: 10.4324/9781003193289-3

Introduction

Community art therapy practice is rich and complex, as both an approach and a setting. The following chapter offers the experiences of art therapists who share the ways that they practice community art therapy. Each reflection expresses aspects of the grounded theory and beehive model discussed in the previous chapter, providing examples and context for how practitioners, clients, and communities at this moment are contributing to the evolution of community art therapy. In the introductory reflection, I offer my own experiences creating Bloom: Center for Art and Integrated Therapies, LLC, a for-profit business, and its journey to becoming the nonprofit Bloom Art and Integrated Therapies, Inc.

Flowers Bloom in Cycles

Bloom to Re-Bloom

Emily Goldstein Nolan

> It has been my work through Bloom that has deepened my connection to my community. As I have worked through each step of creating, maintaining, and then giving the organization back to the community as a nonprofit, I continue to be in awe of the diversity, strength, and resilience of my neighbors around me.

I started Bloom as a limited liability company with a business partner in April 2012. We set up the studio in a local tannery building that had been converted to creative business spaces as well as music practice studios for the community. I had been seeing clients at a large private group practice and was able to bring those clients with me as we established Bloom. I wanted to create a space that integrated community and clinical practice, and I focused on that as a part of my doctoral research. I also envisioned a place that provided the community with access to quality mental health care through art therapy, and a space for art therapists to practice and feel a sense of belonging. I know that I had felt isolated as the only art therapist practicing in a large group practice with other related mental health professionals. I wanted to create a community for art therapists who collaborated and practiced together.

In 2015, my business partner left to pursue other interests and I continued to develop Bloom on my own, but in collaboration with others. In 2017, Bloom moved to a storefront location on the southside of Milwaukee on the neighborhood's main street. At that time Bloom had added five other therapists who were all independent contractors. Art therapists saw individual clients and families with private health insurance coverage and/or the ability to self-pay for sessions. Bloom also began to contract with state health insurance programs,

WRAParound Milwaukee and Comprehensive Community Service, or CCS, that address child and family needs by literally wrapping comprehensive services around identified children and families. Bloom hosted art therapy supervision for new professionals, supervised graduate interns who led low/no cost community art therapy sessions in the studio as well as in other community spaces. Bloom provided different community art therapy opportunities through many partnering agencies.

In 2019, I was invited by Marquette University's Center for Peacemaking to create an art therapy program in the Milwaukee Public Schools (MPS), as a part of a restorative practice educational program for students who weren't finding success in the traditional school setting. I collaborated with school officials, leaders from Marquette, and other local partners to create an alternative school program called the Success Center. Over time, I developed programs and then brought in other art therapists whose interests and skills were aligned with that program effectively to facilitate it. As a result, Bloom offered opportunities for art therapists to expand their practices and created more art therapy jobs here in Milwaukee.

In 2021, I decided that Bloom was on the path to becoming a nonprofit. The organization had already begun to receive grant money through our contracts with MPS, was providing art therapy for free to the community and could be eligible for more grant money to compensate for that work, thereby making Bloom even more sustainable. By 2022, Bloom was established as a nonprofit, and a lot of changes happened all at once. Therapists who were paying practice fees as contractors became percentage employees, creating a shift in how they received their money each month. This change increased Bloom's income to fully cover the costs of what it took to employ the therapists. The first model did not have long-term sustainability, and the change caused a lot of hurt and resentment for some of the therapists who had been at Bloom for several years. The therapists had to decide if the financial situation was feasible for their lives, if these changes aligned with their values and they could support the new version of Bloom. It takes a team to run a nonprofit, which is not easy as it requires a lot of flexibility, navigating complexity, and toleration of ambiguity. With almost a complete turnover of staff, Bloom began anew as a nonprofit.

As a nonprofit we are continually working together to build and maintain our own community of art therapists, interns, and employees. Through working with other effective community teams, I have learned that contributing to a healthy community starts with the organization. We all meet regularly to discuss the agency, day-to-day operations, our work with clients and the community, and to make progress toward future goals and programs. We also make time for fun: at least once a quarter we get together outside of work to explore a new art medium, support a local organization, and strengthen our connection to one another through play. The community-building approach at Bloom is highly relational, respecting, supporting, and valuing one another first, with the intention that this positively impacts the art therapy work we do.

My work through Bloom has deepened my connection to my own community. As I have worked through each step of creating, maintaining, participating, and then giving the organization to the community as a nonprofit, I continue to be in awe of the diversity, strength, and resilience of my neighbors around me. I share this as one way that community art therapy is practiced here in Milwaukee, Wisconsin.

In this text, I widen my notion of who my neighbors are to include fellow art therapists and community art therapy participants who practice and engage in artmaking all over the world. The following reflections expand on concepts that are identified in the grounded theory and beehive model as common components of community art therapy practice. Each reflection is a rich resource and written with an authenticity that demonstrates the complex work that happens when art therapy is practiced in the community.

Making Something Out of Nothing

The Intersection of Art Therapy and Education: Creating Liberatory Practices Within Public Schools

Rochele Royster

> **This type of making and doing was something radically different for them. They didn't know how to respond. For the first time, someone wasn't telling them how to do something or how what they were doing wasn't the right way. It was a new way of working, learning, and being in relationship with each other.**

When I was a young girl, my great grandmother died, leaving me a box of unfinished patchwork pieces that had been neatly folded, pieced, hand ironed, and stacked away in an old shoe box. My great grandmother was a quilter among a list of other things, and I grew up under her quilts. I remember cold Virginia nights sleeping on a handmade bed of layered quilts during family holiday trips. The heaviness of the quilt made it hard to wriggle, toss, and move. The topside was a cornucopia of colors and textures. She had assembled old shirts, dresses, and jeans into a magical tapestry filled with story and song. The underside of the blanket was always an old cotton feed bag. After emptying the feed for the farm animals, she would use cotton sacks for the underside of the quilt. The quilt was heavy with history and burden, joy and laughter, and I remember sleeping so soundly under its weight. A wife and mother in rural North Carolina, my great grandmother had no choice but to be resourceful. She could make a meal out of leftovers, a bushel of freshly picked greens and a hambone, and feed her family and the additional stray mouth that always seemed to be at the table. Her steam-filled kitchen was the liveliest place in the house: her grown daughters and *their* daughters and their men and their boys scurrying about and claiming space filled with laughter or tears or worry. It was a good place to be and observe, evaluate, and learn how to make something out of nothing. It was the backbone of her being and her way of finding and sharing joy.

I transferred that knowledge of quilting and community into my own practice as an educator. After graduating with a degree in studio arts and special education, I went into the classroom. I immediately realized that I did not have the skills to address some of the behaviors I was juggling with. How do I create a safe space conducive to learning that also supports academic growth, emotional intelligence, and wellness? I believed that community-based art therapy could help me create a space within the institution of public schools that could transform our ideas around education, disability, and standardized education and assessment.

My first class was in a small school on the West Side of Chicago. I had 15 students who had been placed in a classroom for students with learning, behavioral, and emotional needs that were not met in the regular education classroom. The students' diagnoses ranged from autism to traumatic brain disorder to specific learning disorder. Many of the students were functioning at least three to four grades below in reading and math. Although they were in 6th grade or above, they were still learning phonics and decoding strategies. Students would often act out during academic instruction. The acting out was a way to mask their deficiencies, eradicate their boredom, or hide their shame in not being able to engage with or understand the learning task and/or lesson. Anger, defensiveness, bullying, and violence were symptoms of larger systemic issues that ricocheted from one issue to another. Issues such as poverty, homelessness, food insecurity, abuse, shame, and illiteracy caused daily burden and long-term trauma. Each day was a new discovery on how to manage behaviors so that I could teach them to read and write. One day, frustrated with the fighting, I decided to turn my classroom into an art studio and gave them the directive to build something. They surely wouldn't be able to fight and throw chairs if their hands were full of tape and cardboard. I gathered random materials I found in the old school: milk crates, a stack of old national geographics, newspapers, fabric, and tape. I removed the rows of desks and created a circle within the room where I carefully placed the found objects. At the beginning of the morning, the students filled the room. They sat at the desks, forced to look at each other within the circle.

"What are we doing today, teach?" Curiosity buzzed and filled the room. "We're going to build something," I said. My comment was met with nervous laughter and confusion. "Build what?" another student asked.

"Whatever we want." I shrugged.

There was a silence that I hadn't heard before. I waited to see who would do what. Would my chair-thrower be the first or the last to pick a material?

The student that never talked and smelled of bleach each morning because she washed all of her and her siblings' clothes in the tub each night before school—how would she interact?

"Where should we begin?" I asked. Silence.

"Any ideas?" Silence.

"What should we make?" Silence.

This type of making and doing was something radically different for them. They didn't know how to respond. For the first time, someone wasn't telling them how to do something or how what they were doing wasn't the right way. It was a new way of working, learning, and being in relationship with each other.

"We can use the tape to hold everything together." I took the tape and started to bind the cardboard together.

Finally, someone spoke. "What if we make a bird."

"A giant one. As tall as the ceiling. So tall, it looks like it might break out."

And then it began. Someone took the tape from my hand and asked for help. I think it was my chair-thrower.

"Hey, hold this here and I'll tape it." Someone responded and they began to build something out of nothing.

That class worked on the bird sculpture for most of the semester. It was huge and yellow and stood in the middle of the class. It had a large beak and wings. It looked like it might just take flight and fly out of there; out of this little forgotten classroom within this under-resourced school sitting on the outskirts of the projects on the west side of Chicago. Other students from other classrooms would peek in and instead of making fun of the special education class, they asked if they could join.

"Can I join this art class?" one student asked. I remember my chair-thrower quickly said "NO! It's just for us. You got to get special permission." He guarded the space. He became the gatekeeper and leader.

We used the bird and the metaphor it represented in our reading and writing. Students wrote stories about the bird and then read their stories to each other. They created characters and imagined what it would be like to fly away; to get out of this cage, this forgotten isolated concrete block. The bird image led us to the story and image of Sankofa, a Ghanaian word that means *retrieve* and is accompanied by the Adinkra symbol represented by a bird with its head turned backwards while its feet face forward carrying a tiny egg in its mouth. This symbol teaches us that we must reach back and gather the best of what our past embodies, so that we can achieve our full potential as we move forward. Our original metaphor of a bird escaping its cage transformed into one that stands tall, learns the best from its past, and moves forward giving back to its own. It became not about the escape but about the recovering, recouping, researching, and remembering. The bird honored the journey, critical introspection, and the application of what had been learned. It was the praxis—a lesson that became part of our collective lived experience through a cycle of action, reflection, and action. Our bird project was our vehicle of expression, connection, imagination, and change. This new transformation was revolutionary—the impetus to conversations about race, education, classism, poverty, and gentrification. How has our history shaped us and how do we move forward with the knowledge we have gained?

At the end of the year, this classroom of misfits, fighters, and loners became a close-knit family that really cared and looked out for each other. I was thankful I was given the academic autonomy to create a transformative space that gave my students the freedom to ask for help, to be vulnerable, to imagine, to lead. Community art therapy created cohesion and trust within a group that was isolated by anger, mistrust, and hurt. The artmaking did not erase the traumas and hard feelings but gave my students the ability to explore these feelings in a safe space using art action to redefine and establish a sense of self outside of the tropes they had adopted or been assigned and to work toward a common goal of caring for each other.

Looking back, I wonder if those lessons were sustainable? How did the process of artmaking impact the larger community? The school in which the bird was created and lived for many years is no longer a public school. The school was closed by Arne Duncan in 2008 as an effort to improve public education with greater school choice. It has been proven a failure. The projects that used to sit behind the school have now been demolished. The building now houses a private college prep school that sits on the edge of the University of Illinois-Chicago campus. The neighborhood in which Martin Luther King slept in to protest work wages and dilapidated housing has now successfully been gentrified. A Costco sits across the street where empty lots and abandoned trash and cars used to be. There are no projects and no community. There is no bird. Where does this process live or sustain itself, if not in a home, or a building, or a scattered fractured community?

One of my former students befriended me on social media almost 20 years after we first met in a classroom. She enjoys crafting and making things like putting words and images on coffee cups and wine glasses. She makes the ordinary items in her life special. I see her often on social media and always respond to her pictures. I saw her the other day in person, and after we exchanged common chit chat, she said, "All these years later, I still do art and make things to deal with my feelings and tough times. You taught me that." And so, that is where *it* lives and where *it* is sustained. It lives in our bodies. In our recipes. In our crockpots and in our kitchens. It lives in our bones and in our hearts and in our work. A life of lessons of process, story, reflection, and action, like a box of old patchwork patches passed on from one artist to another, it lives in our children and their children's children. And repeat.

This singular experience shaped my pedagogy as a teacher and art therapist within public schools. The bird project, sprouted from a greater need, allowed me to understand the importance in building community art/mutual aid projects which can create a radically different classroom and educational experience for students and how they view themselves and their abilities within crisis and/ or community. What do we hope for in education and therapy? What is possible in our classrooms for our youth to create emancipatory and critical spaces that empower their communities? How do we meet our own and each other's needs when the systems and institutions fail us or do us harm? We must create spaces of learning based on a shared commitment of dignity, care, and radical joy. Making something out of nothing—finding joy and comfort despite crisis, dysfunction, and chaos. Transforming birds into Sankofa and carrying those lessons within us as we move forward collectively in connection with each other.

Crafting a Community of Care

Lauren Leone

> **This flow between self- and collective care, growth, empowerment, and action has a reciprocal relationship with a sense of belonging, connection, and agency. Individual and community concerns, self-care and community care, individual identities and voice contributing to a collective message can all be seen in our group, and the craft of quilting is an excellent metaphor for this. A quilt is made of individual pieces that come together to create a whole, without negating or diluting individual contributions.**

Dominator culture has tried to keep us all afraid, to make us choose safety instead of risk, sameness instead of diversity. Moving through that fear, finding out what connects us, reveling in our differences; this is the process that brings us closer, that gives us a world of shared values, or meaningful community.

(hooks, 2003, p. 197)

Crafting Change is a community art therapy craft activism group that has been meeting since September 2017. It began as an eight-week participatory action research project that was part of my doctoral research, and—over four years later—we continue to meet and create together. In this reflection, I'll focus on how collaborative craft has served to build capacity, community, and belonging in our group, including how the community of care we cultivated during the two and a half years we met before the COVID-19 pandemic manifested during the pandemic.

The Group and Setting

The group has a core of eight participants—all of us identify as women and we range in age from late-30s to early-80s; five members of the group are elders. We're a culturally and racially diverse group, made up of African Americans, Afro-Latinas, an Asian Filipina, and one white person (me). One group member's first language is Spanish, and she's been in the process of learning English while our group has been meeting. I've also been working on my Spanish skills outside of our group so I can better communicate with and translate for her in our group. We meet at a community health center in the Roxbury neighborhood of Boston, Massachusetts. While Roxbury has a rich cultural history, including jazz clubs and public art, as well as a long history of grassroots community organizing, the neighborhood has also been impacted by poverty, community violence, and gentrification.

Although I worked as an art therapist at the community health center for several years before the group started meeting, I was no longer employed there in 2017, when the group formed, so in several senses, I'm an outsider to the community. Due to my positionality as an outsider who holds dominant social identities, I found a list of questions that Talwar and Wallis (2021) developed, related to an ethic of care for "collaboration, community art therapy, and social practice," to be important and to help me reflect on this work. They consider:

> What is consent and the power of language? How is the project centering the voices of the community? Who benefits from the project? What is the risk of harm to those being represented by the project or participating in the project? What policies and systemic view does the project address?
>
> (p. 252)

The answers to these questions are fluid, as is community art therapy, which is dynamic and complex.

Community art therapy is grounded in well-being and a strengths-based approach that moves beyond individual clients to focus on "encouraging people to support one another and giving power back to the community. A community model strives to engage many people with the goal of changing the environment, which in turn has a positive impact at the individual level" (Ottemiller & Awais, 2016, p. 148). Community art therapy also aims to instill "in participants a sense of personal and collective agency through expression and feelings of belonging and purpose while furthering healthy connections within the group" (Nolan, 2019, p. 178). In that sense, Crafting Change operates as a community art therapy model in several ways.

First: participants name, negotiate, and share power, and all decisions are made by consensus. We've created a deliberate focus on mutuality and try to engage in solidarity and respect, rather than charity (Lakshmi Piepzna-Samarasinha, 2018).

Second: even though I'm a licensed mental health counselor, and a registered, board-certified art therapist, my role isn't to lead the group; rather, I fluctuate between being a researcher, facilitator, collaborator, advocate, and witness. I participate in crafting and decision-making and sharing skills.

Third: we don't follow a medical model of focusing on individual issues, pathology, or diagnoses but instead focus on well-being and examining issues at a community level. We use critical dialogue circles to engage in self-reflexivity, discuss our projects, and the larger goals of the work we're doing and our individual roles in it.

Part of this self-reflexivity for me is identifying my white, Eurocentric biases and working to unlearn them through ongoing accountability work—as well as noticing when dominant art therapy paradigms may show up in my work and challenging them. I work to subvert the tendency of craft activism to center white women's work. Instead, we look to Black women's art including the story quilts of Harriet Powers and Faith Ringgold, the quilts of Gee's Bend, and projects by the Social Justice Sewing Academy. Grounding our work in culturally resonant materials, methods, and social issues has been an important foundation from which our creative projects have built. In sum, Crafting Change has developed a culture of community care and empowerment that manifests in our collaborative craft projects.

Our Projects

Our group has worked on three major projects in the last four years. The first was a collaborative quilt, *Wake Up Everybody*, part of a participatory action research project using arts-based research to explore the therapeutic potential of craft activism. Participants decided to create a quilt because they felt connected to the strong tradition of African American quilting and had memories from their youth of family members quilting and teaching them to embroider. The aim of this quilt was to bring attention to the gentrification and displacement taking place in Roxbury, as well as a call to viewers to get involved in the housing justice movement. We organized a traveling exhibition of the quilt to disseminate its message. You can learn more about the details of this project in my previous writing (Leone, 2018, 2019, 2021).

Our second project was creating a book of photographs entitled *Crafting Change: Finding Our Way Together* that documented the *Wake Up Everybody* quilt and served as another way of amplifying our message. The book included photos of each participant's contributions to the quilt as well as photos and bios of each participant so that the creators of the quilt weren't nameless and faceless, and we held a crowd-funding campaign to raise funds for the printing costs. Access the photo book at: https://crafting-change.laurenleone.com

Work on our third project was interrupted by the pandemic but we are close to completing it. This project, entitled *The Hidden Figures Dinner Party*, is another collaborative quilt, made with embroidery and appliqué. It pays homage to women and gender nonconforming people of color who have inspired group members through arts, politics, sports, social justice, and/or community organizing. Participants have embroidered 25 portraits so far, and we continue to collect names to be embroidered onto the quilt. Throughout our process, we've discussed each of the potential portraits to include, leading us to tell stories, build knowledge, and share with each other about each proposed honoree's accomplishments and the significance they hold for the individual who suggested adding them to our quilt. This has also allowed room for healthy disagreement and discussion. The group believes this quilt has educational potential beyond our group and we've discussed reaching out to schools and youth-oriented community programs once it's complete. We've also discussed making our quilt even more mobile by creating another photobook and/or a website that would link to biographies and information about each included individual.

The Impacts of COVID-19

I can't tell the story of our group without reflecting on how the COVID-19 pandemic has impacted us. I'm writing this in January 2022. Our group was supposed to meet today but couldn't because of the current Omicron variant surge in Boston. Not only would meeting be unsafe, but the community room we usually meet in is being used for a vaccination booster clinic.

This wasn't the first time the pandemic prevented us from meeting. Our group didn't meet from March 2020 until September 2021. During this time, many people across the world moved work, socializing, entertainment, and even therapy to the Internet; there was an assumption that life could continue online. But, due to the "digital divide," this wasn't possible for our group. Some members of the group wouldn't have been able to join an online group because of barriers to access and literacy with technology created by age and income.

But even though we didn't meet in person for over a year, we still found ways to maintain contact and engage in community care throughout. We spoke on the phone and texted to check in with each other. Early in the pandemic, we offered to drop off groceries and checked to make sure everyone had masks. I mailed fabric and elastic to a participant who was sewing masks to send to her sister in New York City, who was passing them out in her neighborhood which was greatly impacted by the virus. I also mailed a book of poetry by Alice Walker to one participant who was hospitalized, as her favorite pastime is reading Black women's poetry. We checked in on each other when George Floyd was murdered and again when the uprisings took place in response. We shared plans about voting in the 2020 election, news of new grandchildren, and provided emotional support when people were ill. In the spring of 2021, we shared vaccination information and checked in to see if anyone needed a ride or for an appointment to be scheduled. Just last night, one group member texted the group to share information about municipal funds for basic needs assistance.

Although we weren't working on our quilt project, we were still actively engaged in the practice of maintaining community and caring for each other, perhaps in an even more real way than previously, given that we all were sharing a collective trauma that impacted us individually as it also impacted our communities. But as a group, we don't all hold the same level of risk in the pandemic based on what Kimberlé Crenshaw has referred to as the "the intersectional vulnerabilities that twin pandemics lay bare" (AAPF, n.d.) including, among other intersections, of race, class, age, and dis/ability, a topic we've discussed together. Now that we're meeting again, we've resumed our quilt project, but with a new perspective and what seems like a renewed gratitude for our group.

Even in advance of completing our current quilt, we've already discussed plans for a new project informed by how communities of color have been impacted by COVID-19, in general, as well as directly by one participant's experience of hospitalization over the last year. Her identity as an elder Black woman impacted her experience and has motivated the group to focus our next project on health disparities and inequity in healthcare, and advocacy for Black people and people of color in the health care system, especially in building skills for self-advocacy. This idea continues our practice of having our projects arise from discussion about the needs and experiences of individuals in the group and how they reflect larger social issues. This also shows how our group focuses on community and mutual support.

Craft, Community, and Care

Textile artist Claire Hunter (2019) describes community sewing projects as having "emotional and metaphorical currency … [they] are imbued with the spirits of the disparate people who create them, witnessed by others, as unique investments in, and registers of, community worth" (p. 183). This is congruent with the experience of the Crafting Change group when we've exhibited our work; in a community model of art therapy, we've also found that collaborative craft activism builds participants' capacity to address social issues and that developing these skills also serves a therapeutic function (Leone, 2018). Over time, themes such as solidarity and mutuality; belonging and community; and agency and re/awakening have emerged from our work together, reflective of how Talwar (2019) described that "social and community models of art therapy support concepts of belonging and well-being as a collective endeavor" (p. 183). This flow between self- and collective care, growth, empowerment, and action has a reciprocal relationship with a sense of belonging, connection, and agency. Individual and community concerns, self-care and community care, individual identities and voice contributing to a collective message can all be seen in our group, and the craft of quilting is an excellent metaphor for this. A quilt is made of individual pieces that come together to create a whole, without negating or diluting individual contributions.

Similarly, our group has been able to move from banal "we're all equal" approaches to an approach that names and respects the diversity within our group—one that ultimately recognizes that these differences contribute to our community-building because it's "not just what we organically share that can connect us but what we come to have in common because we have done the work of creating community, the unity within the diversity" (hooks, 2003, p. 109).

Quilting has long been associated with community and storytelling, and even sharing skills. In our group, collaborative quilting itself can be seen as an embodiment of a community model of art therapy in that it challenges individualism. In this sense, collaborative craft supports both individual and community realities, and can support us in advocating for social change. In fact, craft historian Glenn Adamson (2021) explained that American craft history "tells us to refuse the false choice between individual and community, to see in craft a unique connection between these apparently opposing values" (p. 316) and went on to describe how craft "has stood right at the junction between individual and community" (p. 314).

This is the third time I've written about Crafting Change for publication. Each time, I've asked participants what they'd like me to share about their experiences of our group. Despite our efforts to tell our story collectively, this reflection is still being told from my perspective and I feel ambivalent about writing about our group for academic audiences. I take to heart Norris et al.'s (2021) reminder that: "The creative arts therapies have a long history of writing about Black clients without Black people. Foundational assumptions and assessments about working with Black peoples and within Black communities are framed through the white gaze" (p. 2). I also deeply resonate with Talwar's description of trying not to "fall into 'romanticizing' a community-based art therapy practice" (2019, p. 180) because I recognize that this group has become tremendously important to me personally—but that doesn't mean that things always go smoothly, and I have to remember that the potential for harm is always present. We are still "finding our way together" which is something for which I have deep gratitude. In the words of Brenda, who we affectionately refer to our as "forewoman" because she keeps us all in line, "The group has come together as a family ... I don't think that would have been possible without the art therapy piece, but [art therapy] is only a piece of what goes on here" (Leone, 2021, p. 173).

References

African American Policy Forum. (n.d.). *Under the blacklight.* https://www.aapf.org/blacklight

Adamson, G. (2021). *Craft: An American history*. Bloomsbury.

hooks, b. (2003). *Teaching community: A pedagogy of hope*. Routledge.

Hunter, C. (2019). *Threads of life: A history of the world through the eye of a needle*. Abrams.

Lakshmi Piepzna-Samarasinha, L. (2018). *Care work: Dreaming disability justice*. Arsenal Pulp.

Leone, L. (2018). *Crafting change: Craft activism and community-based art therapy*. Doctoral dissertation, Mount Mary University. http://www.worldcat.org/oclc /1035718897

Leone, L. (2019). Crafting change: Craft activism for community-based art therapy. In H. Mandell (Ed.), *Crafting dissent: Handicraft as protest from the American Revolution to the Pussyhats* (pp. 247–262). Rowman & Littlefield.

Leone, L. (2021). *Craft in art therapy: Diverse approaches to the transformative power of craft materials and methods*. Routledge.

Nolan, E. (2019). Opening art therapy thresholds: Mechanisms that influence change in the community art therapy studio. *Art Therapy: Journal of the American Art Therapy Association*, *36*(2), 77–85. https://doi.org/10.1080/07421656.2019.1618177

Norris, M., Williams, B., & Gipson, L. (2021). Black aesthetics: Upsetting, undoing, and uncanonizing the arts therapies. *Voices: A World Forum for Music Therapy*, *21*(1), 2.

Ottemiller, D. D., & Awais, Y. J. (2016). A model for art therapists in community-based practice. *Art Therapy: Journal of the American Art Therapy Association*, *33*(3), 144– 150. https://doi.org/10.1080/07421656.2016.1199245

Talwar, S. (2019). *Art therapy for social justice: Radical intersections*. Routledge.

Talwar, S., & Wallis, R. (2021). Quilting across prison walls: Craftwork, social practice, and radical empathy. In L. Leone (Ed.), *Craft in art therapy: Diverse Approaches to the transformative power of craft materials and methods* (pp. 241– 256). Routledge.

Community Art Therapy in Hong Kong

Ling Cheun Bianca Lee

What I ultimately learned on my journey is that community art therapy in Hong Kong is about working with who and what is already there. As art therapists working locally, we must honor the needs of the population by designing, planning, and sharing art in ways that would be accessible to the people. Additionally, I learned to remain critically aware of the role decolonization and intersectionality play in creating projects and collaborations that are mutually beneficial for the HKAAT members and larger local community in Hong Kong.

As an art therapist born and raised in Hong Kong, receiving my undergraduate and graduate education in the United States readied me to face the challenges of adapting to a new art therapy practice when I moved back in 2015. I was immediately flung back into the culture that I once knew with a newfound passion and framework of decolonization and intersectional approaches to share art therapy with my people. Ultimately, besides pursuing a conventional private practice where I meet with individuals and groups providing art therapy in a private studio space, I also developed a community art therapy aspect to meet with more people who have limited access. The journey came with its own trials and tribulations, which I will detail in this reflection on my community art therapy practice in Hong Kong.

However, I must briefly contextualize Hong Kong's local art therapy field for a more comprehensive representation of the population I serve. Hong Kong was a small fishing village prior to becoming a British Colony in 1842. Over the years of British rule, Hong Kong flourished and became the bustling metropolitan portrayed frequently in pop culture. In 1997, Hong Kong transitioned to China's Special Administrative Region when Britain transferred the sovereignty of Hong Kong back to China. From that day onwards, increasing sociopolitical tension continued to build and eventually erupted recently in this Special Administrative Region (Yeung, 2020). This historical overview is paralleled by the push and pull between internalized colonialism (Baskin, 2020) and traditional Confucian values shaping the Hong Kong Chinese identity (Yeh & Yang, 2009).

The development of art therapy in Hong Kong was a pared-down version of the external sociopolitical, cultural, and historical context. We are currently going through our own evolution of shedding the colonial roots and localizing art therapy by developing praxis that best serves our local community. However, there are hurdles that keep us from anything that is equivalent to the Western understanding of the field of art therapy. First, due to low mental health literacy, the stigmatization around mental health care is strong within the Hong Kong community. The public understanding of mental health care often defaults to crisis management and activating high levels of care. Secondly, there has yet to be a licensure system, which is one of the ways any community members or organizations can start becoming more aware of this profession. Finally, the current research and theories of multicultural applications in art therapy are filled with gaps (Talwar, 2018) that do not meet or support professionals who do not practice in the Western context. These challenges reflect ways to manage beyond what a few art therapists can do on our own.

The labor of sharing best practices and education modalities with qualified professionals to the public is dependent on the Hong Kong Association of Art Therapists (HKAAT). The current professional member base includes approximately 35 art therapists who have returned from their master-level training in the West. With the unity of this modest membership base, the challenges seemed more manageable especially when I was elected to step into the role of becoming the president of HKAAT (2017–2021). This position, in addition to my private practice, allowed me the luxury to experiment and take leaps to expand the definition of community art therapy in Hong Kong. Besides the more conventional routes of organizing conferences, publishing the first Chinese language edited book 《藝療藝瞭》, and showcasing the best practices and research of Hong Kong art therapists as a part of the Hong Kong Association of Art Therapists in 2021, my team and I channeled much effort into creating opportunities for the public to access the mental health benefits of artmaking in the community setting.

I developed programming and collaborations with the critical understanding of Hong Konger's intersectional identities, as well as the current systemic, cultural, and sociopolitical stressors (Lee & Au, 2019). These projects all share similar objectives to actively address ways to decolonize the Western-centric knowledge (Singh, 2020) and localize community art therapy practice in Hong Kong. We aim to raise awareness of art therapy, increase people's access to the benefits of the arts, and destigmatize mental health care. By aligning these objectives with local community organizations and resources, I share with you some major projects I have been honored to lead and work on.

The Snow Art Therapy series was created when I was approached by a local mall who put together a "real snowy wonderland" for the public to enjoy as a marketing solution. This is a novel idea since Hong Kong is in the subtropics and local people never experience snow. I proposed an opportunity to allow more access to such new experiences by incorporating community art therapy in the project as a way for the mall to give back to the community. I proposed to facilitate a series of snow art therapy workshops by inviting school-aged community members from underprivileged neighborhoods to participate. These workshops allowed groups of participants to enjoy the facilities, but the snow art therapy workshops supported and contained the narratives and emotions inspired by working with the snow and simple decorative materials.

Since art therapy straddles the arts, mental health, and wellness fields, I collaborated with local wellness and art fairs to make art therapy more accessible to the community in more casual settings. DeTour is Hong Kong's largest design festival that happens annually. The pilot series was named "The Heart Experimentation Lab," featuring artful happenings facilitated by many local qualified art therapists. In a large studio space covered from floor to ceiling by kraft paper, participants in these events added colorful imagery that reflected topics from self-care to one's inner-world exploration. During other visiting hours, besides the happenings, gallery visitors witnessed the evolution of the space as the days of the festival went on. This kraft-paper–clad studio became a physical manifestation of the internal transformation and collaboration among community members who participated. Besides the DeTour, which was more art- and design-centric, I also collaborated with the annual IRIS Wellness Festival. While much of this festival features physical health and wellness, I suggested highlighting the emotional and mental health element through a parent–child community art practice named "HeArt Connection." A dozen guardian–child dyads participated in the artistic collaboration through body tracing and thoughtful sharing to explore the caregiver–child relationship. At the gallery tour of completed artworks at the end, the collective held space for each group member to share their artistic creations with the group using words, gestures, and sounds. The causal setting of the outdoor festival became much more intimate through the sharing that happened in the session; guardians and children found common ground and accumulated more positive experiences together beyond their usual context. These examples exposed a wider community to art therapy and were important steppingstones to realizing larger-scale projects that spanned the city.

Wai Yin Association, a local charity institute that supports and organizes philanthropic projects and events across Hong Kong to those in need, invited me to develop a series of art therapy workshops servicing older adults living in ten different low-income neighborhoods. Within the year of art therapy workshops, the participants experimented with ways they can use art as a conversation-starter and method for stress relief. Not only did the participants benefit from learning ways to incorporate art into their mental health routine, the nonprofit organizations that hosted these workshops were also exposed to the creative arts therapies; as a result, many started to incorporate creative therapies as a part of their programming. This program reached over 1,000 participants, who all gathered for a wrap-up charity showcase honoring all the volunteers, participants, and organizers of the project. The opportunity to meet and connect with many community members through this project enforced my commitment in rising to meet others through art especially in times of need.

In 2019, Hong Kong experienced months of social unrest due to the sociopolitical tension arising from citizens' response to the changing political landscape sparked by the amendment to the extradition law (Lai et el., 2020). The Hong Kong community witnessed frequent violent clashes between the police and protestors. Members of the community continued to move through areas of the city with damaged public furniture, shattered glass at train stations, and posters filled with propaganda from all points of the political spectrum. In response to such traumatic events and stress-inducing environments, I organized a team of volunteer art therapists to provide support groups to community members who were affected by these events. In addition, I initiated an online project named #ArtRechargeHK after seeing how "doom scrolling" affected others' and my own mental health. This online project provides a growing visual library of self-care submitted globally and made accessible to the Hong Kong community via social media platforms. These are only some highlights of the projects I have personally been involved in to promote and share art therapy, which, in Hong Kong, is still ongoing and evolving with the times.

The projects I shared in this reflection all strive to promote the best practice of art therapy for Hong Kong by creating opportunities for the public to access the arts through communal experiences, and potentially bridging those in need with the services that may best fit them. What I ultimately learned on my journey is that community art therapy in Hong Kong is about working with who and what is already there. As art therapists working locally, we must honor the needs of the population by designing, planning, and sharing art in ways that are accessible to the people. Additionally, I learned to remain critically aware of the role decolonization and intersectionality play in creating projects and collaborations that are mutually beneficial for the HKAAT members and larger local community in Hong Kong.

References

Baskin, C. (2020). Contemporary indigenous women's roles: Traditional teachings or internalized colonialism? *Violence Against Women*, *26*(15–16), 2083–2101.

Lai, F., Hall, B., Liang, L., Galea, S., & Hou, W. (2020). Socioeconomic determinants of depression amid the anti-extradition bill protests in Hong Kong: The mediating role of daily routine disruptions. *Journal of Epidemiology and Community Health (1979)*, *74*(12), 988–994.

Lee, B. L. C., & Au, R. W. Y. (2019). Mediating the cultural boundaries: Rise of the lion rock spirit in Hong Kong women. In S. Hogan (Ed.), *Gender and difference in the arts therapies: Inscribed on the body* (pp. 84–98). Routledge.

Singh, A. (2020). Building a counseling psychology of liberation: The path behind us, under us, and before us. *Counseling Psychologist*, *48*(8), 1109–1130.

Talwar, S. (2018). Beyond multiculturalism and cultural competence. In S. Talwar (Ed.), *Art therapy for social justice: Radical intersections* (pp.3–16). Routledge.

Yeh, K. H., & Yang, K. S. (2009). *Chinese filial piety: Psychology analysis* [in Chinese]. Chongqing University Press.

Yeung, B. (2020). *Hong Kong's 2019–2020 social unrest: The trigger, history and lessons*. World Scientific.

Access Art

A Model of Community Care

Angela Lyonsmith and Melissa Raman Molitor

> Once we established an avenue for delivering art materials and accessible arts engagement to children and families throughout the city, we were in a position to develop meaningful ways to address social-emotional needs and provide opportunities for young people to respond to the social, political, economic, and medical crises impacting their physical and mental health.

The Access Art Initiative in Evanston, IL is the outcome of a city-wide response to the emergence of the COVID-19 pandemic in the spring of 2020. Organizations, school districts, local businesses, educators, mental health practitioners, social service agencies, artists, and residents were called upon to participate in a collaborative effort to identify and activate resources to address the immediate challenges faced by the community at large. As art therapists living, working, and raising families in Evanston we experienced the onset of the pandemic on various levels, and our positions as cisgender, able-bodied women with mid to upper socioeconomic status, one of whom identifies as White and one who identifies as Asian and Pacific Islander, informed how we participated in this collective call to action.

Evanston is a university town located to the immediate north of Chicago. The community has a politically progressive reputation that coexists with significant socioeconomic disparity and stark racial divides. Its recent heralding as the first city in the United States to enact a reparations program, and its widespread attention for the equity and racial justice work being done in our local school district, creates an outfacing narrative that is often incongruent to the reality caused by deep historical trauma experienced by racialized communities and the harm that continues to exist. As experienced throughout the country and the world, the pandemic has impacted people in our community in disparate ways and brought to light the existing inequities that have been disregarded for far too long.

Due to our established relationships with Evanston schools through our work as artists, educators, and art therapists, we were able to work directly with the local school district to identify several urgent needs spanning necessities for health and safety, to accessible resources for online schooling and social-emotional support. As a result of the shelter-at-home mandate, school supplies and art materials for children to participate in virtual learning at home was a necessity. A widespread need existed for virtual programming to support children and families during non-school hours. The systemic inequities were again highlighted by the lack of access to resources and support disproportionately affecting our low-income families and Black, Brown, and Indigenous communities the hardest. Our response was two-fold: 1) to get art materials into the hands of children and families in need of supplies, and 2) to create free arts engagement activities and virtual social-emotional programs that were accessible from home.

Access to Art Materials

To address the need for art materials and supplies, we formalized partnerships with local organizations to conduct a donation drive to collect new and gently used art materials and redistribute them to families throughout the city. Individuals and organizations responded to this call with generosity and immediacy allowing us to assemble and allocate over 1,000 free art kits that were packaged and delivered alongside district-wide supplemental food and supply programs.

Engaging in strategic partnerships with organizations and service agencies that had already established relationships with children and families throughout the community allowed us to directly reach those with the highest degree of need.

Their existing knowledge of the children and families also allowed us to tailor the art kits to specific ages, abilities, and interests. For example, our partnership with a local social service agency that supports adolescents, prompted us to design a kit that included fibers, sewing supplies, and materials for mask-making and creative journaling; whereas our partnership with a local tutoring program for elementary school children induced us to provide varying wood pieces, glue, and both 2D and 3D collage materials. From the beginning, we were mindful of the materials we were collecting and distributing. For example, securing crayons and markers that included the "multicultural" skin-tone colors, and including English and Spanish language descriptions. Our material choices became increasingly intentional, and there were even cases where we were able to fulfill requests for certain materials based on what students had at home or what they were interested in exploring.

Access to Virtual Resources

To shift all students to online learning, the city and school district had to address the inequitable access to Internet services that were necessary to allow every student to participate; thus, one of the city's action items was to ensure all students had access to the Internet. Maximizing this increased access, we developed an online platform to deliver various forms of free arts engagement activities, aligning it with the model of asynchronous learning that schools were implementing district wide. The resource was filled with how-to videos, art tutorials, links to artist talks and virtual museum tours with varied levels of complexity for toddlers through teens, and many encouraged collaborative artmaking with others in the home. We were intentional about addressing the need for increased representation and visibility in the content we shared, centering Black, Brown, and Indigenous artists as sources of inspiration for artmaking and presenting how-to videos and guides. Activities included a wide variety of self-directed artmaking using common household materials, recycled materials, organic matter found in nature, and basic traditional art supplies. This virtual resource was updated regularly and shared through school and library e-newsletters, city-wide announcements, social media channels, and word of mouth.

From Basic Access to Meaningful Intervention

The Access Art Initiative was a direct response to immediate basic needs identified by existing community structures. The goal of our involvement was to help grow the collective response and identify the resources and skills we could bring to the table to best support those actions. Once we established an avenue for delivering art materials and accessible arts engagement to children and families throughout the city, we were in a position to develop meaningful ways to address social-emotional needs and provide opportunities for young people to respond to the social, political, economic, and medical crises impacting their physical and mental health.

We began by linking the art kits and online material to increase the potential of these resources. We provided project ideas and tutorials for artmaking that involved materials provided in the kits. We attached QR codes to the art kits to be scanned using a smart phone and those were directly linked to the projects on our site. We explored different tools and approaches that utilized media and technology as a way to dovetail what was naturally happening with increased use of online platforms and virtual learning.

As the pandemic progressed, so did the isolation and separation from social interactions and support systems. To remain connected to the world outside of the mandated shelters, the marked increase in time online led to more hours spent on social media and news outlets. Not only were young people grappling with social isolation and the loss of daily routines and milestone rituals, they were also inundated with constant reports of growing risks to their safety and rising death counts, witnessing real-time racial violence, videos of hate crimes, inhuman political rhetoric, and a surge of overt white-supremacist activity. In an effort to respond to the growing need for social-emotional support and mental health intervention, we expanded our virtual presence to include art-based resources and creative approaches to addressing and responding to young peoples' questions about the pandemic, racial violence, protests, and political movements, and created virtual spaces for adults who are raising or working with children and adolescents to share their experiences, resources, and support.

As more systems were put in place to address the continued needs resulting from the COVID-19 pandemic, our partnerships multiplied. We were able to continue working with existing service providers to identify and address the growing needs through collaborative efforts and alliance building. This allowed us to enact projects and interventions as a form of community care with various groups of people, a few of which are described below.

Virtual Outreach Programming

Using the model of art material distribution and online arts resources, we were able to create free synchronous virtual programs that allowed us to interact directly with people in the community. We sought to replace summer programs for young people that were canceled due to the pandemic, with free virtual art programming, as well as develop online gatherings for people of all ages seeking connection and support. These programs gave us an opportunity to not only supply art materials to people in our community and link them to our online resources, they allowed for direct engagement with them and the development of meaningful interactions and conversations facilitated by the materials we apportioned and online tools we had established. For example, our partnership with a local organization serving families experiencing barriers to social supports and resources, resulted in a six-week online summer art program for elementary school children. In direct response to the height of media coverage of ongoing

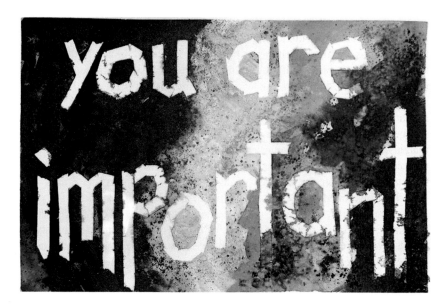

Artwork created in the 2020 virtual summer program

racial violence and glaring social inequities during summer 2020, the program focused on Black empowerment. The art kits and online discussion centered the work of prominent and local Black artists and artists whose work explores equity and social justice as inspiration. The young participants were invited to share their own experiences and perspectives using art and story as they navigated what can only be referred to as the dual pandemics of COVID-19 and racism in our community and beyond.

Another example of our online outreach was a virtual gathering of women who identified as Asian, South Asian, and Pacific Islander (ASAPI) to share their experiences of living and raising families in Evanston amidst the rise in anti-Asian hate and violence taking place across the country. In this case, the model we developed of delivering materials and supplies for individuals to have for the virtual gathering included food and drink items rooted in ASAPI cultural traditions of welcoming and hospitality, art materials, and a printed list of cultural, medical, and mental health resources for local ASAPIs.

Multimedia Care Centers

With a desire to reach young people who were experiencing additional levels of inaccessibility to materials and services due to lack of shelter during the height of the pandemic, we partnered with a local agency that directly serves families and individuals experiencing homelessness in our community. Several local hotels offered temporary housing throughout the summer of 2020 and the agency expressed the need for supplies and activities for kids and families quarantining in hotel rooms. With a line of donation collection already in place, we were able to expand our asks to include items identified by the agency and combine them with their existing donations to create family "activity centers" in the lobbies of the hotels. Although this was a direct extension of the art kit drive, it evolved into an expanded form of outreach as the activity centers grew to include new and gently used games, puzzles, art supplies, books for all ages, and toys for imaginative play. The activity centers were designed with access to sitting areas to encourage interaction while maintaining plenty of space for safe-distancing protocols. The centers were organized by age, ability, and interest, and all of the materials were carefully considered to include books authored by or centering the stories of Black, Brown, and Indigenous, and toys and art materials that were accessible for various abilities and skill levels. In an effort to preserve elements of dignity and joy, the centers were presented with care, staged as free shops with welcoming signs and restocked weekly, and whenever possible we endeavored to secure items that were requested by the families.

Evanston Art Connects

The city of Evanston has a strong arts foundation, and local artists and arts organizations played a significant role in maintaining community connection during the peak of the pandemic. We worked with many of these artists and organizations to organize a community initiative entitled Evanston Art Connects—a citywide call for residents of all ages to create and display art in windows, doorways, yards, parks, and on causeway trees, sidewalks, and storefronts. This could take the form of ephemeral murals of chalk art to elaborate participatory installations. Themes ranged from gratitude for health care professionals and essential workers, to graduation messages for students reaching milestones during quarantine, to Black Lives Matter and #StopAsianHate activism. The art kits we distributed at this time supported equitable engagement in this widespread initiative and were stocked with relevant supplies. A local arts organization created a digital map containing locations of all the artwork on display to encourage people to get outside for a "gallery walk" or take a drive to view the community installations. We posted documentation of the art, activism, and symbols of hope created by makers of all ages on social media in an effort to increase engagement and we also shared them on our evolving virtual platform.

***

The Access Art Initiative, and its evolution into several forms of creative outreach and community care, was rooted in sustainability as it relied upon redirecting resources already present in the community to meet collective needs. The initiative increased accessibility of the arts and artmaking for all community members and allowed families to engage with broader resources while still in the midst of social distancing measures. The initiative allowed us to focus on how we might use our sphere of access and knowledge to address the needs identified by the community at large. We were able to apply our expertise related to designing art kits and virtual resources that were accessible, developmentally informed, and supportive of social-emotional needs while also offering some much-needed distraction, creative engagement, and fun during the height of the pandemic and political unrest of 2020. We addressed the needs identified by the community in ways that allowed us to draw on our personal and professional practices that center equity, social justice, sustainability, and a strengths-based approach to care. What began as a crisis response has since developed into a formalized nonprofit organization called Kids Create Change. Our work continues to be grounded in community partnerships and collective care as we create spaces and develop programs that use the arts to center the voices and stories of people who are marginalized due to their social identities, and who experience barriers to accessing the arts, social-emotional support, and cultural experiences grounded in resiliency, hope, and change.

Recognize, Reimagine, and Restore

Reflections on Cultural Humility Within Community-Based Art Therapy
Louvenia Jackson

> **When is silence aligning with injustice? When do we move beyond silence and self-preservation to voice activism? Collectively, with other art therapists and those interested in culturally informed art therapy research, I have looked at these questions to address the ways art therapist use art/creativity to understand our internal experience (Silence), connect with community (Solitude), and voice inequality (Solidarity).**

Identify in Silence

We recognize in silence; within our solitude, we reimagine; with solidarity, we restore. Community is solace.

The summer of 2020, while supervising students in virtual artmaking groups, I observed a session in which a young black man in attendance shared his lived experience related to *silence* in response to the prompt of that day. He shared that for him silence was necessary during that time (social justice demonstrations following George Floyd's death, months dealing with the pandemic, and the acts of the administration of that time). He said, for him, silence was necessary because there was so much noise, that he needed quiet. And how he appreciated coming to the art therapy sessions where he had the time to sit in the silence of his artmaking without having to hear the "noise."

That struck me, and I continued to reflect on silence, solitude, and solidarity. I wanted to further explore that idea of silence. What arises in times of silence? What does silence mean to each individual? What is collective silence? How do we interpret silence? And how do we all relate to it culturally, and in what ways? I was interested in exploring and researching this during the time of COVID-19. I was motivated to seek meaning. And in this search, a call for the end of silence through advocacy, public awareness, collaboration, and interdisciplinary partnership. And in that, as an art therapist, art therapy educator, and national presenter, I wanted to bring attention to the events of 2020 and the voices that were marginalized and the communities impacted.

As I continued to contemplate, I realized that it wasn't just silence that was significant during this time, but it was also the solitude that was brought on by the social distancing of the pandemic. The solitude that many sat in because their voices were not heard, their communities were being oppressed, and their bodies harmed. And how many people during the pandemic were alone and experienced that aloneness in so many ways? Then it brought me to the idea of solidarity and how the silence may have exacerbated issues of equity and belonging. And how silence also could have been a way to preserve and protect us during those moments of harm. How solidarity is entered and experienced because of the ways different people perceive silence. When is silence interpreted as solitude, and when is it an act of solidarity? And how all those considerations determine how we connect to one another, how we perceive one another, how we can sit in understanding. How we can hear and amplify voices that are not being heard. How do we help those who feel isolated, disenchanted, disregarded, or discarded? How do we use the privileges that we have to create change?

When is silence aligning with injustice? When do we move beyond silence and self-preservation to voice activism? Collectively, with other art therapists and those interested in culturally informed art therapy research, I have looked at these questions to address the ways art therapists use art/creativity to understand our internal experience (silence), connect with community (solitude), and voice inequality (solidarity).

Reimage Within Solitude

The first step in community-based art therapy is outreach and visibility. Many projects I engage in come from being approached by members in the community who have seen or heard of my work and enquire, with a need for support. During the pandemic, many communities impacted by isolation, fear, and pain were seeking ways to connect with others and communicate their personal and collective trauma. Without access to others, together with the community-based organization (CBOs) I needed to think of creative ways to get the arts to these communities. This required mailing materials to registered virtual participants, providing materials at community spaces for virtual participants to pick up, and offering ways for them to engage with whatever materials were available to them in their own spaces. We searched for free online creative platforms and offered links and tutorials. This reimagining expanded access to services and ways to practice community-based art therapy.

Connecting with the community requires many steps and considerations. During the initial contact with the community-based organization (CBO), I learn about the community by asking what has been used, what is effective, and how I might support them. I communicate from a collaborative perspective. Once a mutual relationship is developed, together we begin the planning and start with the preparations. Each person takes on tasks and roles that align with our skills and capabilities. Together, the organization and I identify and develop a team. Once the team is introduced and informed, ideas and suggestions are solicited from all members before moving forward. The next step is identifying outcomes, objectives, and strategies to meet shared goals. After the team has dialogued, the art project is developed based on that collective information. Once the art project is agreed upon, together with the training and education of the art therapist and the expertise of the community, the team discusses what prompts to use and how to acquire materials. This collaborative effort means determining the financial resources available and how to make the project equitable for all members involved. The community art prompt can align with the collective goals. Next, the implementation of the project is developed. Often at this point there can be planning challenges. The structure frequently must change with the needs and limitations of the community and the availability and the flexibility of the art therapist. Details of the planning are important and impermanent; they help guide all those involved. The program needs to have the elasticity to move with the community as they experience challenges and growth. This can come in the form of a plethora of community artmaking, from free drawings and portraits, collage to mural, and sculptures to mosaics. The importance is that it comes from the voices of the community and can be supported by the art therapist. At the end of the artmaking experience the community must consider thoughtful plans to present the completed project. It is a way to involve all members, as well as share the experience with the larger community. It becomes a celebration and marker of time and space. It welcomes and communicates the importance of the art experience as well as how the community can move forward with similar endeavors. It can inspire and motivate. The aspect of community work that can be difficult and often missed is the evaluation of current and future resources. The community-based effort is most impactful if it can be sustained. One way is to evaluate its effectiveness and assess the outcomes. Collecting data helps with the debriefing and the dialog about the next steps. It also offers a foundation for research that can support future endeavors. Accountability at all these steps gives structure and opportunities for financial stability for the community and community-based art therapy education training.

> The arts also allow communities to retrieve traditional cultural forms that may have fallen into disuse, and thereby strengthen social networks. These are intermediate steps for both individuals and communities who are involved in processes of moving from silence towards transformative action.
>
> (Watkins & Shulman, 2008, p. 239)

Restore With Solidarity

Art therapists need to recognize the importance of finding strength and particularly finding strength within defined communities that have been silenced and retold through the narratives of others. Many communities are treated as if disenfranchised and marginalized by the way they are depicted and described as being without internal resources or lacking ability or strength. In a sense, the terms *disenfranchised* and *marginalized* might be accurate when looking at these communities as being *underserved*. From another perspective, they can be seen as endurable and able to bolster themselves in many ways. Part of the work of the art therapist when engaging with the community is understanding the importance of partnership. The third principle of cultural humility states, "developing mutually beneficial partnerships with communities on behalf of defined populations" (Murray-Garcia & Tervalon, 1998). The strength of an art therapist is understanding the importance of allowing the community to be the expert of their own lived experience and being with the community through a collaborative process to help with their needs, whatever those needs may be. "Art therapy must endorse and promote community-based art therapy as a way to move the field into the future, where community practice becomes paramount in addressing the stress and development of mental health challenges before, they reach our office" (Jackson, 2020, p. 88). One can choose a community and a community can choose us. Communities can enhance our growth and stifle our goals. The development of community is comprised of personal contributions along with collective knowing.

> We are chronicling the link between how we memorialize collective history and how we experience personal history, how silence and suffering in one realm may reproduce silence in another. Authoritarian structures in the family and individual mirror those in the political world. Amnesia in the political realm can reinforce silencing in personal life. The retrieval of memory and self-expression through the arts can disrupt such a system.
>
> (Watkins & Shulman, p. 236, 2008)

Before going into a community, art therapists must critically assess why we have decided to go. Whose needs are we trying to meet? It is important to know that a community's needs may not come from a place of inadequacy but from a place of oppression, a place of being stifled, a place where one is not able to flourish and grow because of needs not being met. These are the challenges of defined communities. Not the fact that they *can't*, but the fact that they are *not able to*, because extenuating factors make it difficult for them to thrive. As art therapists we need to be attuned to those considerations and offer a partnership to understand the wisdom that already lies within communities.

A way to extend upon the third cultural humility principle of mutually beneficial engagement with community is to support an open environment. The art therapist is open to being corrected as a facilitator, willing to own their mistakes, and acknowledges the members of the community in their work and what they have brought to the space. We can see ourselves as superior to other disciplines, skills differences, and education, instead of acknowledging that we are all here for the same cause and everyone has something to contribute. Art therapists working with the community must value input from all perspectives. This requires using an emic versus an etic approach: emic meaning collectively learning from within all cultures, allowing our practice and research to be informed by this collaborative perspective; as opposed to etic, where our knowledge comes from the outside and the perspective of others. Having a "both/and" view, where emic and etic is used thoughtfully, can offer a balanced approach. Everyone is an expert in their discipline and role; everyone can be a teacher or expert, no matter what level of education or experience.

COVID-19 highlighted the impact that communities can have on government, education, and health. Many efforts these institutions attempted were challenged if they did not have the backing of communities. I believe that in recognizing the importance of community, art therapy is now moving toward a community-based model. This can have more of an impact on the individual because of the relationship to community, and foster equity in services and approaches. Cultural humility offers a model of critical self-reflexive practice to prompt ways art therapists engage with others and the community. The art therapist with cultural humility understands the importance of community mutual collaboration, which begins with self-reflection and ends with accountability, both for self and institutions. Just as there is a delicate balance in cultural humility, so there is a balance between personal and collective perspectives (Jackson, 2020, pp. 146–147).

In finding the balance of cultural humility, I believe art therapists can become community art healers along with other healers within communities that have passed down and continue to revive, inspire, and invigorate their spaces/ members through art. Together with communities we can reimage, rebuild, and restore. Watkins and Shulman (2008) speak about liberation art projects as engagements in the rebirth of solidarity, which can cause social cohesion and community-building, with facilitators of liberation arts projects restoring the connection between power and freedom, speech and silence, building new myths and solidarity for the future. "Cultural workers who help organize community liberation arts projects … are community healers or cultural therapists who help repair the fabric of community life" (Watkins & Shulman, p. 241, 2008). Art therapists—let's expand our awareness and identities by recognizing community-based work, reimagining our roles within community spaces, and restore the relevance of collective art healing in art therapy.

References

Jackson, L. (2020). *Cultural humility in art therapy: Applications for practice, research, social justice, self-care and pedagogy.* Jessica Kingsley.
Tervalon, M., & Murray-Garcia, J. (1998). Cultural humility versus cultural competence: A critical distinction in defining physician training outcomes in multicultural education. *Journal of Health Care for the Poor and Underserved, 9*(2), 117–125.
Watkins, M., & Shulman, H. (2008). *Critical theory and practice in psychology and the human sciences: Toward psychologies of liberation.* Palgrave MacMillan.

The Value of Digital Community in Art Therapy

Gretchen M. Miller

> The power of technology creates dynamic possibilities for community-based considerations related to enhancing relationships, communal engagement, and mutual aid. The ongoing use of digital communities in art therapy is an essential landscape to bring individuals and groups together to decrease isolation, find support, and a sense of belonging.

Fostering community through technology has become an embedded form of life vital to our daily communication, relationships, activities, and engagement. What debuted during the Internet's beginning history of using electronic bulletin boards, listservs, newsgroups, chatrooms, and web forums (Chen, 2019) has now given way to highly interactive, dynamic, and immersive forms of digital communities. The contemporary use of digital community in art therapy leverages sophisticated platforms for global professional engagement, collaboration, obtaining continuing education, academic learning, providing art therapy to clients, as well as a valuable means for activating and sustaining creative practice (McDonald & Miller, 2020; Miller, 2018; Miller, 2016).

Values and Benefits

Digital communities embrace values that promote egalitarianism, participatory culture, as well as equity and inclusion (Collie et al., 2017; Gerity, 2010; Humphreys, 2016; Rodgers, 2011). Individual members are regarded as valuable co-creators to the community to help assist one another and benefit the whole group, despite varying levels of experience, education, skills, or expertise. This shift away from hierarchal structure adds to the digital community's open and rich exchange of shared knowledge, resources, and ideas. "Art therapy students, new professionals, practicing art therapists, seasoned experts, and retirees from all around the world can collectively access and engage in opportunities to advance their art therapy practice or studies" (Miller, in press). These values also encourage and create mutual accountability to each other and within the overall digital community.

In my book *The Art Therapist's Guide to Social Media*, (Miller, 2018) I included some reflections from Dr. Harriet Wadeson that described the reality of art therapists as "often working in isolation from other art therapists" (1995, p. 14). This separation, according to Wadeson, often removed the art therapist from opportunities to discuss and share ideas with another colleague from an art therapy lens. Now, a plethora of digital communities and access to online networks with art therapy professionals from around the world are easily and readily available on our mobile devices, tablets, and laptop computers to mitigate experiences of disconnection. Wadeson also recommended that art therapists managing isolation participate in conferences and workshops to boost needed support and relational connection to art therapy. At the time of Wadeson's writing (1995) this was only possible through physically attending events and gatherings. Technology has made this form of engagement much more accessible and equitable to participate in. Virtual opportunities for meeting together have removed some of the financial, travel, location, and time barriers associated with attending in-person events. Art therapists have many choices to connect through social media, webinars, online courses, workshops, and conferences, as well as virtual art studios to engage with art therapy colleagues regionally, nationally, and globally. This aids in building inclusion, strengthens belonging, and increases resilience through communal support and meaningful relational connection online (Miller, 2018). Virtual spaces can also support individuals, groups, and communities during times of crisis, displacement, loss, and adversity. The coronavirus pandemic is one recent example of how digital communities can be mobilized and leveraged in art therapy to sustain relationships, a sense of belonging, as well as to amplify hope and connection (Miller, in press; Miller & McDonald, 2020; Potash et al., 2020).

Community Care

Nakita Valerio, an award-winning writer, researcher, and Muslim community organizer based in Edmonton, Canada recently put the value of community care into the spotlight. After horrific mosque mass shootings in Christchurch, New Zealand that murdered 50 Muslim worshippers, (Mahmud, 2019) Valerio took to social media and posted that we fail people by telling them to take care of themselves when what is really needed is taking care of each other through community care. Valerio's post quickly spread through social media and went viral on many platforms among the online community (Dockray, 2019; Valerio, 2019)

Self-care, as most widely known, is an individually focused practice that is viewed as an act of compassion directed toward oneself to take care of our own well-being. This form of self-care sends the message that if *you* want to feel better, *you* are responsible for doing the labor yourself, for yourself. Self-care is often an individual solution for a collective problem, offering only temporary, isolated relief for deep-rooted structural and systemic issues that people and communities face. On the other hand, community care centers on the collective. The core value of community care unites individuals to mutually help and support one another, emphasizing the reciprocal exchange of resources and services for the shared benefit to empower people through solidarity instead of charity. Community care also provides an opportunity to work together on repairing wounds and the factors that created them though navigating and addressing social issues and systems collectively (Dainkeh, 2019).

Art therapists can empower community care online. Art therapists can use their creativity and art expression to share messages of compassion, support, hope, and affirmation through acts of creative kindness. For example, I created the Creative Deed Project where I created a mini piece of art every day and then abandoned the image in physical spaces such as gas stations, the post office, at work, on the campus where I teach, on car windshields, in elevators, grocery stores, and many, many more places. I also posted my creative deeds online, created a social media group to invite others to create and exchange creative deeds, and activated a project hashtag, #creativedeed365 to help locate some of the creative deeds people discovered when they shared them online. "Small groups in various communities around the globe formed around this creative task, creating art, sharing adventures of selfless giving, and providing support to one another along the way" (Lorenzo de la Peña, 2018, p. 33).

Art therapists can also engage in digital activism and advocacy through art-making and creative expression. Digital advocacy is the use of technology to bring awareness to and organize individuals or groups of people to take action around an issue or cause (Bowen Ray & Schlehofer, 2014). Art therapists engaging in activism and advocacy often use dialoguing and community-building through art to create social change (Potash, 2011; Vance & Potash, 2021). To translate this into a digital space, art therapists can activate their creativity and art expression online to bring attention to social justice issues and to organize virtual community-based projects, calls for actions, digital petitions, campaigns, toolkits, and can use intentional, socially engaged hashtags.

Art therapists can also contribute to creating a culture of community care in online spaces that are welcoming, value belonging, and foster collaborative engagement. We can commit to helping make digital spaces feel safe, inclusive, and an environment where ideas and thoughts can be freely or openly expressed and exchanged. Art therapists can be mindful of the energy we bring into online spaces, giving special attention to how to support, affirm, and dialogue with others in this shared environment with humility. In digital spaces, practitioners can remember to slow down their social media responses, taking time to pause and bring awareness to their intention behind participating in online spaces as well as the power of their impact before choosing to publish and contribute to online posts and comments (Miller, 2018). Creating safe spaces online also includes making digital communities accessible. Art therapists can be aware of and empower different learning styles, abilities, and levels of energy that can impact participation. We can integrate diverse ways to communicate content and information online that use video, images, subtitles, or captions, alt text descriptions, as well as digital tools and applications that can enhance accessibility and universal design.

Conclusion

As this reflection has addressed, the power of technology creates dynamic possibilities for community-based considerations related to enhancing relationships, communal engagement, and mutual aid. The ongoing use of digital communities in art therapy is an essential landscape to bring individuals and groups together to decrease isolation, find support, and a sense of belonging. Opportunities for connection, community, and creativity exist through global virtual spaces and will continue to provide opportunities for empowering inclusivity, artmaking, safe spaces, and coping for art therapists and their clients.

References

Bowen Ray, H., & Schlehofer, M. (2014). Using social media for digital advocacy. Center for community health and development. University of Kansas. https://ctb.ku .edu/en/table-of-contents/advocacy/direct-action/electronic-advocacy/main

Chen, R. (2019). The history of Internet communities. [Medium Post]. Retrieved from https://medium.com/@rchen8/the-history-of-internet-communities-f0234db848b1

Collie, K., Prins Hankinson, S., Norton, M., Dunlop, C., Mooney, M., Miller, G., & Giese-Davis, J. (2017). Online art therapy groups for young adults with cancer. *Arts and Health, 9*(1), 1–13. https://www.doi.org/10.1080/17533015.2015.1121882

Dainkeh, F. (2019, December 30). Beyond self-care: Understanding community care and why it is important. She+ geeks out [Blog post]. https://shegeeksout.com/beyond-self -care-understanding-community-care-and-why-its-important

Dockray, H. (2019, May 24). Self care isn't enough. We need community care to thrive. *Mashable* [Blog post]. https://mashable.com/article/community-care-versus-self-care

Gerity, L. (2010). Fourteen secrets for a happy artist's life: Using art and the Internet to encourage resilience, joy, and a sense of community. In C. Hyland Moon (Ed.), *Materials and media in art therapy: Critical understandings of diverse artistic vocabularies* (pp. 155–182). Routledge.

Humphreys, A. (2016). *Social media: Enduring principles.* Oxford University Press.

Lorenzo de la Peña, S. (2018). Reminiscing on building communities through creative deeds. *Australian and New Zealand Journal of Arts Therapy, 13*(1 & 2). https://anzacata .org/resources/Files/11_ANZJAT/ANZJAT-2018/8.ANZJAT-2018-SLP-a.pdf

Mahmud, F. (2019). New Zealand mosque attack: Who were the victims? *Aljazeera* [News Report]. https://www.aljazeera.com/news/2019/3/22/new-zealand-mosque -attack-who-were-the-victims

Miller, G. (2016). Social media and creative motivation. In R. Garner (Ed.), *Digital art therapy: Material, methods, and applications* (pp. 40–53). Jessica Kingsley Publishers.

Miller, G. (2018). *The art therapist's guide to social media*. Routledge.

Miller, G. (in press). Art therapists and digital community. In M. Winkel (Ed.), *Virtual art therapy: Research and practice*. Routledge.

Miller, G., & McDonald, A. (2020). Online art therapy during the COVID-19 pandemic. *International Journal of Art Therapy: Inscape, 25*(4), 159–160. https://www.doi.org /10.1080/17454832.2020.1846383

Potash, J. S. (2011). Art therapists as intermediates for social change. *Journal of Art for Life, 2*(1), 48–58.

Potash, J. S., Kalmanowitz, D., Fung, I., Anand, S. A., & Miller, G. M. (2020). Art therapy in pandemics: Lessons for COVID-19. *Art Therapy, 37*(2), 105–107. https:// www.doi.org/10.1080/07421656.2020.1754047

Rodgers, K. E. (2011). Virtual communities as egalitarian societies: Why contributions matter and what they mean. Anthropology Department Theses and Dissertations. 17. https://digitalcommons.unl.edu/anthrotheses/17

Valerio, N. (2019, April 16). This viral Facebook post urges people to rethink self-care. https://mashable.com/article/community-care-versus-self-care

Vance, L. D., & Potash, J. S. (2021, October 7). Black lives matter protest art: Uncovering explicit and implicit emotions through thematic analysis. *Peace and Conflict: Journal of Peace Psychology* [Advance online publication]. http://doi.org/10.1037/pac0000584

Wadeson, H. (1995). *The dynamics of art psychotherapy*. John Wiley & Sons, Inc.

Letting Lived Experience Lead

Reimagining Community Arts and Community Art Therapy

Allison Tunis

> With education and positions of power often more accessible to people with privilege, many programs are led by people who do not fully understand the experiences that community members are faced with and ultimately cause further harm by perpetuating systems of oppression. To truly change the outcomes and allow for community healing and thriving, the systems need to be restructured. This involves every one of us in the community reflecting on where we fit in the system, how we contribute to the system, and how together we can break free of the oppression.

Over the course of the last decade, I have facilitated a variety of community arts projects and programs with a diverse array of people and populations. Even though I always focus on mental health–related programming and healing from trauma, some of the groups I work with are communities that I am a part of and some groups I only narrowly overlap with in experience. One of the most important takeaways I have had from these experiences, and from the education provided by my peers along the way, is that the people whom we as art therapists serve in community arts—clients, participants, and any other euphemisms often used to separate "us" from "them" in traditional hierarchies of practice—these are the people who should be developing and leading the services that are targeted towards them—in community arts, community art therapy, and beyond. This doesn't mean that one must match up identically with a community to collaborate with them. However, it does mean that art therapists need to be working to restructure practices to be more "user"-driven, less hierarchical, and more accepting of lived experience as expertise. This process is required from conception to completion in order to make space for more diverse and authentic voices and to support the success of the community, while causing as little harm as possible.

One way to enact this is to have more people with lived experience (experiences that are in common with the community being served, as well as experiences from intersecting identities and groups that have been marginalized or are seeking equity) in positions of power—which include the positions of creating and facilitating community arts projects and art therapy programs. As a person with multiple intersecting identities myself, some marginalized and some privileged, I have come to greatly appreciate the value there is in having shared lived experience when facilitating programs and providing care to community. Through the experiences I have had with different communities, I have come to understand the strengths I bring and where I need to collaborate with others. The participatory nature of collaboration ensures that the communities I serve are supported to inform and control their own care and be provided care that meets their needs appropriately. This reflection will cover some of the benefits of lived experience–led programs, the hazards of *not* centering lived experience, and how we can start to reimagine systems and practices to put these ideas into action.

Why Should Lived Experience Lead?

A phrase that you may have heard before is "Nothing about us without us." Although originally coming out of political calls for democracy in Poland in the 1500s, it was reclaimed by disability activists in the 1990s (Khedr & Etmanski, 2021). This call highlights the need for the involvement of disabled people in their own care—something that has often been overlooked or intentionally withheld due to implicit biases about the capabilities of people with disabilities and the integration of these biases into our systems of care. When art therapists ensure that people with lived experience, whether it be with regard to disability or other identities, are the ones who are creating and leading the support networks for their communities, communities benefit in several ways. One of the most important ways I have seen is that having people with lived experience creating and leading programs allows for more effective and anti-oppressive care. I spent several years working with street-involved youth, many of whom were living with mental health–related and other disabilities, but who also faced innumerable challenges around poverty, race, gender and sexuality, intergenerational trauma, and substance use, among others. I shared only the narrowest of lived experiences with many of them and found that my work during that time likely taught me more than it taught them—an education for which I am immensely grateful but which I know was likely gained at the expense of the youth I worked with. I was also able to see how important it is to invite leaders with lived experience to work with the community. Many of my colleagues were individuals who had come from similar backgrounds to the youth and the care they were able to provide, coming specifically from a place of knowledge, understanding, and deep compassion, was integral to providing care to young people in crisis. This isn't to say that my contributions were not important but that it was only through the collaboration with and education from other peers with more personal experience that I was able to offer care to the youth I worked with that would meet their needs and work to overcome some of the ways that I personally contribute to systemic oppression. By acknowledging the limitations to what I could offer and recognizing my privileges and implicit biases, I could provide more targeted care and ideally reduce the harm that comes from ignorance or a lack of empathy for the experiences of others.

Another reason why it is important to have leaders with lived experience is to allow for more diverse and authentic representation in our communities. Seeing empowered people like oneself can lead to greater self-confidence and shame resilience—an important consideration in a world that seems intent on telling everyone that they are never enough, but especially those with marginalized identities. In later programs I ran for 2SLGBTQiA+ youth, it was important for me to be open and public about my own identity and to lead by example by being proud and willing to stand behind who I am. I know that as a youth I didn't see many people in my community who were like me—queer, fat, neurodiverse, and disabled—and that made me feel very alone, atypical, and ashamed throughout my life. I also recognized that just one leader wasn't enough—there are a myriad of other identities that I don't possess and experiences I cannot speak to. To address this, I planned for guest facilitators every other month in our program, and invited people from different backgrounds and communities, including the youth themselves on occasion, to lead with the support and resources of the group and to speak openly about their own experiences. Seeing people succeed who share one's identities, especially when they are from communities that have been oppressed or stigmatized, allows others from these communities to see the possibility of themselves succeeding as well. Additionally, when communities are provided representation, more authentic and diverse stories are also heard by those outside of the represented communities. Current systems have made it so that we are exposed to only certain types of content and information, such as through algorithms and social media or through people who are given power and control in our communities. It is only through the sharing of stories from people outside of these privileged and empowered positions that we as art therapists can start to recognize where we have failed or have more to learn, build empathy and understanding, and really grow to provide better care.

What If We Don't Let Lived Experience Lead?

Although there are many benefits to centering people with lived experience and making room for them in positions of leadership, there are also many detriments to *not* doing so. It isn't simply that communities would fail to reap the rewards that lived experience leadership brings, but that by not supporting people with lived experience and gatekeeping positions of leadership, those in power are causing further harm. "One doesn't have to operate with great malice to do great harm. The absence of empathy and understanding are sufficient" (Blow, 2012).

Without people with lived experience in positions of leadership, the opportunities grow for microaggressions and implicit biases to make their way into programs and care, further reinforcing systems of oppression and continuing to keep people at the margins. When those with lived experiences are kept out of positions of power, communities become further divided into "caregivers" and "care receivers," creating an "us" versus "them" mindset. This approach deepens gaps in empathy and reinforces traditional power structures where people who are care receivers do not have a say in, or control over, their own care, and those who do have the control are disconnected from and unaware of the real-life experiences of those they are supposed to serve. By refusing to share the platforms and power we have as art therapists and facilitators, we reinforce the status quo and perpetuate systems of oppression that continue to harm our clients.

Change the Process, Change the Result

What can art therapists and community practitioners do to center lived experience in our practices? Leaders are role models for progress, which often means not only acknowledging one's own limitations, but giving up some of one's own power to create more equitable systems that prioritize collaboration, diverse voices, and compassion. In my current collaborative community arts series working with peers who live with chronic illness, I am working to explore and develop processes that reflect on and incorporate these considerations around power, cooperation, and sharing lived experience.

This project seeks to develop a more equitable and anti-oppressive approach to portraiture and artmaking, specifically focusing on breaking down hierarchies often present in art practices – by listening to and centering lived experience, recognizing and addressing the power differentials between "artist" and "model", and reflecting on questions about elitism and exclusion within art communities, the value of creation vs. concept, insider vs. outsider art, craft vs. fine art, and art ownership and consent practices.

(Tunis, 2021)

Specifically, through this project I am seeking to disrupt traditional artistic practices by merging community arts and art therapy into fine art practices. Further, by rejecting the notion that the artist is the sole creator and instead shares creative control and ownership with the "model" as a collaborator, I aim to build a process where all collaborators are integral and have control over their image and portrayal, in contrast to the historical exploitation of models and marginalized people in art. This is emphasized not only through the collaboration of creative vision, but also by working to make the financial and in-kind compensation for all collaborators equitable and reflective of the labor provided.

To consider as well, there is the specific risk of tokenization that comes along with asking people with lived experience to share their stories. Often, people are asked to "sit at the table," but without any real structural change or compensation (whether financial, in-kind, or other). When art therapists and community practitioners collaborate with people with lived experience, it is integral that supporting and sustaining structural changes and equitably compensating those involved is made the top priority. Compensation for collaboration needs to be built into funding proposals and programming costs, accessibility and intersectionality need to be reviewed and addressed regularly, and receptivity and accountability to feedback cemented into the foundation of all that is done in community. Throughout this project,[1] I have continued to reflect and recognize areas where my practice can be improved by asking myself: "Who is profiting from this work?" The answer should always be the community first and foremost, and then those who are supporting the work itself. By centering lived experience and restructuring to give back power to communities, we ensure that they are the beneficiaries of all we do.

Conclusion

Traditionally, mainstream society has considered those who are able to access specialized education to be experts but forget about the people who are living the experience day-to-day. The individuals who are truly experts on what kind of care is needed are the people who need the care themselves. Especially, but not exclusively, with regard to disabled communities, individuals are often assumed to be less capable of being experts and less capable of leading, when the truth is that there is a wealth of wisdom and empathy that communities can gain by supporting those at the margins to lead. With education and positions of power often more accessible to people with privilege, many programs are led by people who do not fully understand the experiences that community members are faced with and ultimately cause further harm by perpetuating systems of oppression. To truly change the outcomes and allow for community healing and thriving, the systems need to be restructured. This involves every one of us in the community reflecting on where we fit in the system, how we contribute to the system, and how together we can break free of the oppression. Freedom ensures that the programs created and facilitated benefit the people they are created for and not just the people who create them. It is only through actively changing the power structures from the inside out that we can truly begin to disrupt and dismantle the systems that keep disabled people and many others in poverty and powerlessness.

Note

1 The chronic illness collaborative art series is scheduled to be exhibited in 2023 and is supported by the Edmonton Arts Council, the Alberta Foundation for the Arts, the Canada Council for the Arts and the McMullen Gallery/Friends of University Hospitals.

References

Blow, C. M. (2012, September 19). I know why the caged bird shrieks. *The New York Times*. https://campaignstops.blogs.nytimes.com/2012/09/19/blow-i-know-why-the-caged-bird-shrieks/

Khedr, R., & Etmanski, A. (2021, June 17). Nothing about us without us. *Disability Without Poverty*. https://www.disabilitywithoutpoverty.ca/nothing-about-us-without-us

Tunis, A. (2021, November). Untitled chronic illness project 2021–22. *Art from Here*. https://www.artfromhere.ca/artists/allison-tunis

Artist Buddies

A Community of Artists Who Accompany Each Other

Pat B. Allen, Abbe Miller, and Andrea Inés Velázquez Dorgan

> **Even across borders in a virtual milieu, we were able to provide sacred space to one another by holding the intention to invite the Creative Source into our process together, accessing a different level of what is often called "safe" space. Each of us was doing her own work but we felt we were being held together by something greater and beyond ourselves.**

In the spring of 2019, as COVID-19 locked down communities around the world, Judy Lucas, founder of the organization Friends of Fieldworkers,[1] asked for help. The children of the field workers were at home without their parents, essential workers, to help them adapt to school on Zoom. She thought art therapy could help support the children in these conditions. This chapter will describe the birth of "Artist Buddies," an international collaborative project in which trainees in Open Studio Mexico were paired with children in Ventura County, CA, to make art together via the Internet. A unique community of practice developed as the trainees met monthly virtually with the authors, three art therapists, for support, supervision, and our own artmaking. Insights emerged from this practice that help to clarify the unique mindset of community and accompaniment that develops when one's own art practice is centered to guide our work with others.

We claim the broadest definition of "community" in this reflection as we imagine who and what community art therapy can be. A community is a group of people who share some or multiple characteristics. We define this community using the characteristics of those who are inherently creative, who have within themselves the answers they need, and who have something unique and valuable to share with the world. The presence of the word "therapy" implies for us that members of this community have suffered, have experienced loss, and have been challenged as they make their way in the world. Anyone, therefore, is a potential member of this community. The defining characteristic that circumscribes this community is the engagement in artmaking expressly to care for and explore experience on behalf of self, others, and the world. We hold that offering an invitation into this imagined community is the first order of responsibility for a community art therapist. In such a community, the art therapist is an artist, a fellow traveler, and a co-creator of the art experience. Our clinical skills recede in this way of working and our artist self comes forward. In a recent "Reflection on what 'art' does in art therapy practice and research" (McNiff, 2019) Shaun McNiff offered this essential message: "Do the work within the context of your specific community and in your distinctive way, with an openness to how it is integrally connected to the whole human experience" (p. 162). During the past two years many of us have learned lessons about what constitutes our community and especially how we are all integrally connected. We offer here some of the insights we gleaned from a unique opportunity that grew out of the COVID-19 pandemic.

When Judy Lucas, founder of Friends of Fieldworkers, contacted the first author of this piece, she asked for art therapy for children who were home on lockdown due to COVID-19. While parents everywhere were scrambling to monitor and support their children as they transitioned to online learning, the parents of these children, who are essential workers, were expected to keep working in the fields. The children were on their own to figure out how to make do. Judy mentioned that several of the children had a special interest in art. This was the part of her request that resonated. What she was asking for was support, which in her mind was clearly encompassed by the term "art therapy."

The families in question have migrated from Mexico and perform basic agricultural work in low-paid and under-supported conditions while their children make the transition to what they hope will be a more prosperous future with expectations of assimilation into American culture. As the pandemic unfolded, Judy's organization immediately responded to needs in the fieldworker community, providing basic services, such as masks, which employers failed to do. Whatever art might have to be provided would be offered via the Internet. Judy vowed to ensure each child had a device, and Internet access to be able to meet virtually.

I thought immediately of my colleague and fellow author here, Andrea Velásquez, founder of Open Studio Mexico (OSM), which trains individuals in the Open Studio Process (Rubin, 2016). I asked Andrea if perhaps her students might be willing to volunteer to meet with children and share artmaking as an experiment. Andrea coined the term "Artist Buddy" to encompass both the supportive and egalitarian nature of the relationship we envisioned and the neutral quality of what would be offered. Open Studio Process is always about making art alongside others in parallel process, offering companioning in the creative process in co-created spaces. As bilingual individuals, the OSM students would be able to easily circumvent any language issues that might arise. We wondered what sort of cultural interactions might occur between the children who had emigrated and the adult students residing in Mexico, the country the families had left.

The work would be without pay for the students and Andrea felt that offering a parallel process of artmaking and potential supervision would be a fair exchange. Abbe Miller, another author here, had recently completed her doctoral research on the one-canvas El Duende painting process (Miller, 2012, 2020), where individuals continue to paint for multiple weeks on the same piece, documenting changes each time. We wondered if the one-canvas method might be a good suggestion for the Artist Buddies since the children would be working at home and might have limited space. Volunteers from Friends of Fieldworkers supplied materials to the children. Abbe, Andrea, and I would meet regularly online with Open Studio Mexico students who volunteered to participate. We offered this time together as one of inquiry and artmaking where we would hold a space for reflection and support of the volunteers as needed. We would also reserve a good portion of that time for us to make art and try out the one-canvas approach together.

What we quickly learned was how much each of us needed a supportive community of fellow artists during this strange time of lockdown and quarantine. This chapter allows us to just dip a toe into what we learned. Some of the insights are that even across borders in a virtual milieu, we were able to provide sacred space to one another by holding the intention to invite the Creative Source into our process together, accessing a different level of what is often called "safe" space. Each of us was doing her own work but we felt we were being held together by something greater and beyond ourselves. There were moments when concerns arose about the relationships of the students with their artist buddies that called forth our therapist selves. We listened to the inner therapist voice and allayed her fears. In each case we reminded one another that our commitment was to "lead with our artist self" and call the artist self forth in each relationship. Once this happened the therapist self was able to relax, and the work proceeded with ease. We trusted that each one of us was being guided and that our work together brought forth the commonality of our spiritual, artist, and human selves.

Artist Buddies was a modest experiment but provided an opportunity for deep and rich enquiry. A total of five Artist Buddy pairs met for over one year. Our facilitator space met 30 times to make art together. In the words of Andrea: "It felt like we were building a culture," drawing out from each of our creative process what we needed to be fully alive. Each pair of Artist Buddies was unique. In one case, a brother and sister met weekly with a buddy in her sixties. The siblings had emigrated from the same province in Mexico where their buddy was from. They shared experiences including customs to celebrate Día de Muertos. The adult buddy was transported back into memories of her family of origin which she expressed in her artmaking. Concentric circles of care developed as the adult buddies met with the authors and we made art together virtually.

Sharing the designation of artist connected all of us who participated in this project to the children as well as to one another. We found echoes of one another's images arose in unique forms in our artmaking. Sometimes it was a novel use of a material, such as painting over crumpled paper to add texture to a canvas; other times an image, such as a heart, a bird, or a radiant yellow light found its way into multiple art works. The authors and OSM students mostly adhered to the one-canvas El Duende method, photographing each iteration to keep track of how the images unfolded. Having the visual record in an ongoing slideshow also created a shared community of images that we could revisit between sessions. A community of care developed for all of us that made the strange conditions of lockdown and isolation more bearable.

> When art is placed in a central context it cannot be reduced to an adjunctive role, which traditionally has relied on psychological models. Rather, this model draws upon the complexities of art, which can be messy and challenging … pleasure experienced from artmaking can dissipate suffering and pain.
>
> (Thompson, 2010, p. 23)

We found that this shared art process flattened hierarchies and allowed each of us to show up in our full self, our shared humanness, and our existential need for meaning; all these aspects were more apparent during the COVID-19 pandemic as we learned an entirely new way to be together in a virtual, rather than a physically shared, studio space.

The purpose for sharing this novel reflection in a book about community art therapy felt compelling but obscure at first. We seek to lift up the most unique, yet subtle, gift embedded in art therapy—the embrace of an artist's identity. Rilke (1934) wrote,

> To let each impression come and … feeling it come to completion, entirely in itself, in the dark, in the unsayable, the unconscious, beyond the reach of one's own understanding, and with deep humility and patience to wait for the hour when a new clarity is born: this alone is what it means to live as an artist.
>
> (Letter 3)

The artist identity is perhaps what is most vitally needed to weather the storms of change, the birth pangs of the new that the entire world is experiencing. As art therapists, we have the vision to see this world as both a crucible of change and as a beloved community to whom we extend the invitation of artmaking and the artist identity as a way to connect, gain support, recognize the divine within each of us, and make meaning for a shared future.

Note

1 Friends of Fieldworkers, Inc., is a non-profit charity established to befriend, celebrate, and support families of fieldworkers in Ventura County.

References

Allen, P. (2016). Art making as spiritual path. In J. Rubin (Ed.), *Approaches to art therapy* (pp. 271–285). Routledge.

McNiff, S. (2019). Reflection on what "art" does in art therapy practice and research. *Art Therapy*, *36*(3), 162–164. https://www.tandfonline.com/doi/abs/10.1080/07421656 .2019.1649547

Miller, A. (2012). Inspired by el duende: One-canvas process painting in art therapy supervision. *Art Therapy*, *29*(4), 16173. https://doi.org/10.1080/07421656.2013 .730024

Miller, A. (2020). One-canvas method: Art making that transforms on one surface over a sustained period of time. https://digitalcommons.lesley.edu/expressive_dissertations /94/

Rilke, R. M. (1934/1981). *Letters to a young poet*. Letter, 3. Norton.

Thompson, G. (2010). Intermodal aspects of aesthetic space: Phenomenology of self and other. Paper presented at the Expressive Therapy Summit. New York.

The Creation of an LGBTQ Community Art Therapy Practice

Chelsea O'Neil and Owen Karcher

When we first imagined the center, we listed things that felt like freedom. What would it be like to build expressive arts therapies services led by queer and trans people, considerate of the unique traumas our communities face? Bold enough to trust that our people are resilient and that their healing is within reach? In the hopelessness and frustration of our context, we started naming glimmers of possibility.

Tucked into a nondescript shopping complex, the windows of our community art therapy practice display a colorful poster by Micah Bazant that reads, "We all belong here; we will defend each other." Amidst big-box stores and suburban sprawl, transgression and resistance brew, conjuring possibilities and invitations to those on the margins to unravel and exhale. A vibrant, mixed-media mural hangs on a 48" × 48" canvas in the lobby. The response to the directive "using lines, shapes, and colors, what is transgender liberation?" reads, "dignity," "okay, okay, okay, okay," "we are all beautiful," "freedom," "love and support," "gender has no rules," "I am open and safe to bloom," and "light," encapsulated by hand-drawn and painted images of people with outstretched arms, flowers, spirals, and the four elements. At the center, a dove holding a rose represents the demand of trans women of color to "give us our roses while we're here." The art piece, created by clients in asynchronous collaboration, serves as an invitation to hope, which feels vital as transgender liberation can often feel far away. The mural is a symbolic representation of what we created in our practice. The artists never met one another, spanned age and demographics, and their artistic abilities ranged from professional to first-timer. Yet here, on the canvas, in our space, they joined together to represent a thriving community of possibility, a community striving for healthier, stronger, more beautiful relationships and choices for themselves, and the people they love.

Madison, WI, is a city hailed as one of the best places to live in the United States, year after year (Livability, 2021) while also being one of the most racially unequal (Wisconsin Council on Children and Families, 2013). The discrepancy between the thriving and the barely surviving is glaring. Poverty, mental illness, violence, suicide, homelessness, discrimination, over-policing, rejection, and isolation are woven into the LGBTQ experience in Madison. Nationally and locally, our communities face targeted efforts to revoke our rights through legislative attacks and public miseducation campaigns rooted in fear and violence (ACLU, 2020). When the practice began in 2015, clinics offering LGBT-specific services were decreasing (Chen et al., 2021), and marriage equality had yet to pass. While recognition of marriage equality moved some rights forward, the fight fell too often on assimilationist rhetoric and misaligned priorities that alienated and further condemned those of us existing outside normative standards (Spade, 2015). Now, several years later, legislators continue their attempts to legislate us out of existence by criminalizing transgender-affirming healthcare, sports, and education.

As queer and trans practitioners, we acknowledge the ways we are affected and privileged by systems of oppression and are mindful of our sociopolitical locations as they offer us resources, privilege, and limitations of understanding. As a result, we practice in ways that further our education and depth of practice, challenge personal and community collusion with power and structural inequality, cultivate structural competence (Shelton et al., 2019), and develop creatively queered and comprehensive approaches to working with clients (MacWilliam et al., 2019). We honor our clients' abilities to identify an inner calling toward authenticity that is intrinsic in coming to understand queer and trans identities.

Despite what the media or political rhetoric espouses, we proclaim that transgender people are inherently beautiful and healthy, gender deviance is welcome and natural, and cisgenderism and oppression are traumatic.

Although we both came of age in southern Wisconsin, we always felt a tight constriction wrapped around our expressions of gender and sexuality and an overwhelming expectation of homogeneity. The strict confinement of white, Christian, heteropatriarchal dominance can suffocate LGBTQ people, particularly those who stretch the limits and do not, or cannot, assimilate. Black and Brown, immigrant, poor, disabled, queer, and trans people are constantly, passive-aggressively, and violently reminded of their otherness daily. The demands to perform the constriction and neutralization of one's identity to be more palatable are constant and often masked with a liberal facade of "Midwest nice," making it challenging to name.

We wanted to build what we could not find: support and access to care without fear of rejection and stigma. Queer and trans people are continually mistreated and violated by care providers who don't understand or value their identities (Four Corners: TNB Health Research Advisory Network, 2021; James et al., 2016). We sought to build a practice for LGBTQ people of all identities centered on their dignity and bodily autonomy. We hoped to create a model that would interrupt barriers to care and provide guidance for navigating the daunting labyrinth of the medical-industrial complex.

When we first imagined the center, we listed things that felt like freedom. What would it be like to build art therapy services led by LGBTQ people, considerate of the unique traumas our communities face? Could we be bold enough to trust that our people are resilient and that their healing is within reach? Then, in the hopelessness and frustration of our context, we started naming glimmers of possibility. We would have chairs wide enough and strong enough for bodies of all shapes and sizes. There could be blankets and pillows for nesting on the floor! Affirmations will be taped to mirrors and tucked on bulletin boards. Art will fill the walls, and the art supplies will be readily accessible. There will be books filled with stories of LGBTQ people living joyful lives. A sliding scale will open us up to those experiencing financial hardship. We imagined our own needs, and then we added more ways of saying, "You belong here." The list came forth like a spell.

Intersectional (Grzanka, 2014; Talwar, 2019), liberatory (Duran et al., 2008; Watkins & Shulman, 2008), and critical transpersonal approaches (Hocoy, 2005; Hocoy, 2016) provided the scaffolding of our work together and traced back to when we met in graduate school. Our practice was informed by Indigenous activist principles, as articulated by artist and organizer Lilla Watson: "If you have come here to help me, you are wasting your time. But if you have come because your liberation is bound up with mine, let us work together." This quote hung proudly on the wall where we first met as art therapy interns. Our clinical supervisor, Tsunemi Maehara Rooney, planted many seeds that blossomed into our shared dedication to community liberation. Our unique framework was informed by women of color and queer elders at Safehouse Progressive

Alliance for Nonviolence and the Buddhist, transpersonal approaches taught by our instructors at Naropa University.

Our orientation is trauma-informed and rooted in bodily autonomy and sex-positivity. We trust LGBTQIA+ people to make decisions about their bodies rather than creating obstacles to accessing hormones or other life-saving gender-affirming treatments. Unfortunately, these frameworks are not widely held in the mental health field and are not made readily available to the burgeoning number of clinicians in training programs. As a result, many LGBTQIA+ experiences have been pathologized, controlled, neutralized, cleaned up, or shamed. The field of psychology has created harm through pathologization and colluded with larger systems of control to police trans and queer people out of existence (Spade, 2015; Talwar, 2019); this history and the ways current art therapists are conditioned need to be examined and transformed.

To expand the bounds of our context and invite possibility, we returned to the transpersonal teachings we both received as master's students. Transpersonal is defined as experiences of identity or self-extending beyond (trans) the individual or personal (Kaklauskaskas et al., 2016). Queering a transpersonal psychology framework invites spirituality and consciousness beyond the norms of cisgender, heterosexual dominant narratives (Seda, 2021). We witnessed the benefits of merging sexuality, gender, and creativity to push the boundaries of self-expression and develop a stronger sense of self. It is important to name that our practice did not disregard our privileged identities and experiences, a practice known as bypassing. Contrarily, we held a deep sense of responsibility to change environmental conditions through advocacy, activism, formation of relationships, all born in spiritual and contemplative practice. We held ceremonies in our space and invited clients into culturally specific rituals. We cultivated relationships with the land and the plants living on it.

After years of working in places that felt sterile, chaotic, urgent, and dehumanizing, we were determined to create an environment that invited the whole being by communicating ease, choice, comfort, safety, and support. The design of the space was informed by what we called hospitality. Each detail brought into the space intended to signal, "you belong." We chose representative imagery and resources to reduce barriers to comfort; warm paint colors, a non-gendered, accessible bathroom, live plants, sensory fidget toys, and limited scents and sounds for those with sensitivities. These intentional "indicators of safety" consider the ways minority stress (Meyer, 2003) creates anticipation of discrimination and violence and aim to relieve the protective contractions and tensions held in the body. We spent hours thinking about how we wanted people to *feel* when they interacted with us and entered our doors, including people who shared our identities. More importantly, those who had different experiences require us to acknowledge our privilege and make concerted efforts to challenge ourselves to go deeper.

Within the first year of opening the center, people traveled from 61 cities across the state, some driving four hours, to receive counseling. We wrote 60 letters for gender-affirming hormones and surgeries in the first year and 101 in the second. Our clients ranged from ages 4 to 70, individuals and families, couples, almost exclusively identifying as transgender and gender-expansive. Listening deeply, offering reflections, and providing non-judgmental guidance supported our clients in developing healthy coping strategies, setting boundaries, declaring truths, and taking action. When sessions moved beyond talk therapy and into the realm of imaginal and expressive therapies, we were witnesses to new levels of possibility and self-authorship that we couldn't have anticipated.

The art provided a container for self-exploration and play. Our shelves were lined with glittery self-portraits, delicate clay figurines, gender dysphoria embodied in sharp monsters and erratic scribbles, dolls representing anger, anxiety, and joy, and hand-crafted boxes full of wishes for the future. We were all artists, finding meaning and form while trusting an uncertain and beautiful process to unfold. Queerness and transness are rooted in creativity and possibility, imagination, and risk-taking in ways that are beautifully supported by the practice of art therapy.

Today, we can recall profoundly nourishing moments with clients. The wide eyes of a six-year-old trans boy speaking with an adult trans man for the first time! The tears of joy and euphoria in a post-op session. The sigh of relief and awkward laughter that comes when someone first says their chosen name or asserts their pronouns aloud. The 60-year-olds who came to us after decades of delaying care or being refused care, moving swiftly through their transition process with the aid of the network we built, not without challenge but with renewed confidence in the possibility of pursuing their authenticity and truth. The parents who said, "We don't know what to do. Will you help us?" then dutifully brought their children to therapy and trusted us with their care, listening to their children as they drew boundaries or declared pronouns or names and asked for what they needed. Crafting this space was the honor of a lifetime.

Our clients' stories, particularly their art, moved us deeply and fueled a fire in our bellies that demanded action. Sitting across from people in a therapy room was incredibly important, but with a gaping void of services, it wasn't enough to truly, ethically meet their needs. We were determined to build a broader network so that we could facilitate connections to other providers and opportunities for hope and transformation. We needed to bolster our client's support outside of therapy. Fueled by urgency and a deep sense of over-accountability in the face of a destructive system, we did everything we could to improve the climate for LGBTQ people in big and small ways. We trained hundreds of service providers, responded to community crises and calls for community organizing, testified at the city council to ban conversion therapy, wrote op-eds, co-hosted a queer youth book club, and convened diverse practitioners regularly to help clients access resources.

The work in those early years was deliberate, all-consuming, and unsustainable. In fact, we do not recommend taking on the burden of saving all queer and trans people! We do not advise any orientation toward saving, healing, or even helping LGBTQ people as this reinforces a power imbalance that positions clinicians as the expert or rescuer. True liberation and wholeness cannot be offered, prescribed, given, or granted. LGBTQ people are not a problem to be cured, a challenge to be resolved. Our job as clinicians is to join our clients in their inherent wholeness and reflect on what is true and brutal and beautiful about their lives so *they* can make meaning and come out stronger and more prepared for what comes next. It is within a clinician's purview to make a deliberate effort to clear obstacles from that path. We cannot simply witness the pain and offer Band-Aids week after week. As art therapists dedicated to social justice, we must tend to the systems and oppressive elements that wound and re-wound our clients until the violence stops (Hocoy, 2005). We must sit with the pain and hold it tenderly, let it change us, and then do something to prevent the harm.

As we write this, both of us know this can feel daunting, but it is possible. It takes an ongoing commitment to build more connection to our deepest, truest selves while holding space wide enough for the totality of others' fullest, truest selves. This means unweaving the tendrils of internalized oppression and bias *and* creative engagement with the possibilities of liberatory community. It takes acknowledging imperfection, asking for support when needed, and allowing ourselves to be changed in the witnessing of growth and healing. This journey requires the knowledge that we cannot separate LGBTQ liberation from racial justice, feminism, disability justice, anti-capitalism, violence prevention, constructive abolition, and sovereignty because the LGBTQ community is not a monolith. Our stories and possibilities are vast. We are all connected, and we need each other.

References

ACLU. (2020). *Trans rights under attack in 2020.* https://www.aclu.org/issues/lgbtq -rights/transgender-rights/trans-rights-under-attack-2020

Chen, D., Watson, R., Caputi, T., & Shover, C. (2021). Proportion of U.S. Clinics offering lgbt-tailored mental health services decreased over time: A panel study of the national mental health services survey. *Annals of LGBTQ Public and Population Health, 2*(3), 174–184. https://doi.org/10.1891/lgbtq-2020-0071

Duran, E., Firehammer, J., & Gonzalez, J. (2008). Liberation psychology as the path toward healing cultural soul wounds. *Journal of Counseling and Development, 86*(3), 288–295. https://doi.org/10.1002/j.1556-6678.2008.tb00511

Four Corners: TNB Health Research Advisory Network. (2021). *Four Corners: Health Research Priorities among TNB Communities.* https://howardbrown.org/wp-content /uploads/2021/03/FourCorners-HealthResearchPrioritiesAmongTNBCommunities _Final_3_21.pdf

Grzanka, P. (2014). Introduction: Intersectional objectivity. In P. Grzanka (Ed.), *Intersectionality: A foundations and frontiers reader* (pp. X–XXVII). Westview.

Hocoy, D. (2005). Art therapy and social action: A transpersonal framework. *Art Therapy: Journal of the American Art Therapy Association, 22*(I), 17–33.

Hocoy, D. (2016). Transpersonal psychology in the age of ISIS: The role of culture, social action, and personal transformation. In F. J. Kaklauskas, C. J. Clements, D.

Hocoy, & L. Hoffman (Eds.), *Shadows and light: Theory, research, and practice in transpersonal psychology: Principles and practices* (pp. 31–43). University Professors Press.

James, S., Herman, J., Rankin, S., Keisling, M., Mottet, L., & Anafi, M. (2016). *The report of the 2015 U.S. transgender survey.* National Center for Transgender Equality.

Kaklauskaskas, F. J., Clements, C., Hocoy, D., & Hoffman, L. (Eds.). (2016). *Shadows and light: Theory, research, and practice in transpersonal psychology* (Vol. 1). University Professors Press.

Livability. (2021). 2021 top 100 best places to live in America. https://livability.com/best-places/2021-top-100-best-places-to-live-in-america/

MacWilliam, B., Harris, B., Trotter, D. G., & Long, K. (2019). *Creative arts therapies and the LGBTQ community: Theory and practice.* Jessica Kingsley Publishers.

Meyer, I. H. (2003). Prejudice, social stress, and mental health in lesbian, gay and bisexual populations: Conceptual issues and research evidence. *Psychological Bulletin, 129*(5), 674–697. https://doi.org/10.1037/0033-2909.129.5.674

Seda, D. (2021). LGBT inclusivity in transpersonal psychology: A case for incorporating LGBT spiritual experiences in transpersonal education. *Journal of Conscious Evolution, 18*, Article 2. https://digitalcommons.ciis.edu/cejournal/vol18/iss18/

Shelton, J., Kroehle, K., & Andia, M. (2019). The trans person is not the problem: Brave spaces and structural competence as educative tools for trans justice in social work. *Journal of Sociology and Social Welfare, 46*(4), 97–124.

Spade, D. (2015). *Normal life: Administrative violence, critical trans politics and the limits of law.* Duke University Press.

Talwar, S. (2019). Beyond multiculturalism and cultural competence: A social justice vision in art therapy. In S. Talwar (Ed.), *Art therapy for social justice: Radical intersections* (pp. 3–17). Routledge.

Watkins, M., & Shulman, H. (2008). *Toward psychologies of liberation: Critical theory and practice in psychology and the human sciences.* Palgrave MacMillan.

Wisconsin Council on Children and Families. (2013). *Race to equity: A baseline report on the state of racial disparities in dane county.* https://racetoequity.net/baseline-report-state-racial-disparities-dane-county/

Studio and Gallery Practices to Promote Empathy and Understanding

Jennifer DeLucia

Gallery exhibits helped to bridge gaps in understanding and empathy between veterans and civilians by engaging civilians in viewing, witnessing, and learning about veterans lived experiences through their participation as gallery visitors. The range of connections fostered—with the studio, the art itself, and those who viewed the art—helped to reduce the isolation experienced by many veterans during transition.

Veterans experience a transition when they return home from military service and resume life as a civilian citizen, or a resident who is no longer part of the Armed Forces (DeLucia & Kennedy, 2021). This passage from military to civilian life is a largely interpersonal process. It involves social, emotional, and physical changes that take place within the context of relationships with children, spouses, partners, friends, family, and the veteran's broader home community. Consequently, transition is impacted by the psychological state of civilian citizens, and the community, who welcome the returning veterans (DeLucia, 2016). How members within the community take care of one another, how the community responds to difference, and the availability and access to resources are just a few of the factors that may impact the veteran's military-to-civilian transition.

Given the impact that one's sense of home and community can have on veteran transition, it was a significant moment when I heard a veteran refer to the art therapy studio where he was receiving services as his "second home." As a practitioner and researcher, I was curious to explore the needs associated with transition and how the art therapy program where I was practicing addressed these needs. I initiated a participatory action research study aimed at bringing veterans together to contribute to the design of their art therapy program and meet their self-identified needs. In this process, the veterans became researchers. The study design included a series of focus groups involving dialogue and artmaking that supported the team of ten veterans to develop a list of concerns they felt to be pivotal to a successful transition. Participating veterans (herein also "veteran researchers") explored personal experiences with art therapy services and determined ways that art therapy addressed the needs associated with military-to-civilian transition.

Seeking Connection, Understanding, and Purpose

Several veterans acknowledged that they needed to feel physically and emotionally safe to start their transition process back into their communities. They acknowledged that social support, such as family and friends, and some professional services contributed to a felt sense of safety (DeLucia, 2015). Yet many participating veterans perceived their existing support network as unprepared to help. One veteran discussed the experience of trying to talk to friends about combat experiences and described how they would quickly change the subject to something more positive.

Another concern related to social support was what participants identified as incorrect civilian assumptions about their military experience (Caplin & Lewis, 2011; Sayer et al., 2010). Many felt that there was a disconnect between civilian understanding of service and a veteran's experience of service. The absence of this support and understanding often led veterans to withdraw from these relationships. This response was especially concerning given that research consistently attests to the importance of social support as a key factor in successful transition (Caplin & Lewis, 2011; Furukawa, 1997; Larson & Norman, 2014).

Several veterans in the group identified that they sought a sense of belonging, brotherhood, or family, and joined the military for the camaraderie and group cohesion it offered. They felt at home within their own veteran community. For veteran participants who found this level of support and sense of belonging only in the military, the transition out of service was challenging. All participating veterans said they had been changed by their service experiences; some changes were positive, others negative. Regardless of their overall attitude toward their service experience, they had shared concerns about self-identity. As their service commitments concluded, they were forced to reconfigure their identities and senses of purpose.

Sense of Belonging and Community in the Studio and Gallery

The art therapy studio provided a physical space for veterans to connect through artmaking and the veterans art gallery served to address the military–civilian divide by inviting the broader community to experience veterans lived experiences in a new way—through the images and experiences shared in their artwork. Both the studio and gallery provided meaningful ways for veterans to find and contribute to building a supportive community.

Drop-in open studio group sessions helped to ease the social isolation veterans associated with the military-to-civilian transition. Veterans participating in the group often felt an immediate sense of belonging among veteran peers and responded to the veteran-led group structure. During these sessions, the art therapist functioned as a participant-facilitator, creating art alongside group members while working with the group to maintain a safe and welcoming space.

The creative atmosphere of the studio environment welcomed new veterans joining the group. The studio inspired creative risk-taking through engagement with art materials, the physical environment, image-making, and group energy that developed among participants (Allen, 1995; Luzzatto, 1997; McNiff, 1995; B. L. Moon, 2010). A sense of solidarity and comradeship developed among veteran participants who shared workspace and materials. Artmaking served to communicate and share lived experiences among group members, and it helped to foster a culture of support and friendship.

The group sessions served as a way into treatment for some veterans. As they became familiar with the art therapy program, including its philosophy, and practice, they developed a sense of trust that the services were helpful, revealing opportunities to work on more focused therapeutic goals in individual sessions (DeLucia, 2015). Alternatively, the group served as a transition out of individual services for other veterans who engaged with the group to maintain their creative practice and broaden their social network.

A veterans' art gallery was a separate space in the community where monthly art exhibits were held. Gallery exhibitions raised public awareness and understanding of veterans' experiences, while formal art openings endorsed the artwork of veterans by bringing it into the broader art community (see also Howells & Zelnik, 2009). As exhibiting artists, veterans self-advocated and informed the public of their lived experiences, while at the same time expressing and taking ownership of their own perspectives (DeLucia, 2015).

Veteran researchers emphasized that art exhibitions contribute to an affirming and more well-rounded veteran narrative. The gallery space served as an intervention to decrease isolation and disconnection between veterans and the civilian community by bringing the community together in a participatory way for honoring, reflecting, and witnessing the stories, people, and experiences reflected through the artwork on display (DeLucia, 2015).

Community-Based Art Therapy with Veterans

Based on their personal experiences with art therapy and military-to-civilian transition, veterans from the research team identified seven core principles of art therapy, many of which reinforced the need for connection and community, and the ways that community-oriented approaches addressed those needs (DeLucia, 2015). The core principles included that art therapy offers psychological safety, promotes growth, gets to the heart of the matter, builds connections, draws out strengths, cultivates a sense of purpose, and awakens emotions. These core principles were also consistent with many found in the art therapy literature (e.g., McNiff, 1988; B. L. Moon, 2008, 2010; Riley, 2001; Rubin, 2005; Waller, 1993). Although all these core principles are important when working with transitioning veterans in art therapy, for the purposes of this reflection I offer expansion on ones that are particularly meaningful when considering community art therapy approaches.

1. **Art therapy offers psychological safety.** Veteran researchers described how they were able to achieve or find a sense of emotional and physical safety in the art therapy studio. Safety was developed through their participation—by engaging with the art materials offered, creating artwork, and by building relationships among other veterans and staff during the drop-in studio group sessions. The studio itself offered a creative and supportive atmosphere (Fenner, 2012; Henley, 1995). Veterans described the studio as a "loving and caring environment" and "a place that lifts me up." One veteran described the studio as his "safety area," and another as their "second home." Veterans took ownership of the studio space by caring for the materials, attending to cleaning needs in their workspace at the end of a session, and oftentimes by finding a physical space in the studio that became their own—where they left in-progress artwork and materials. Feeling a sense of ownership of the space supported veterans to let their guard down, and by participating in a supportive and caring community they started to address underlying needs, feelings, and concerns related to transition.

2. **Art therapy builds connections.** The main goal of the art therapy program was to build connections among participating veterans and their social supports, as well as the broader community. The studio functioned as a place for veterans to connect with other veterans. Another source of connection was the artwork on the studio walls. The studio was a living space that was filled with veteran artwork, while participants in individual art therapy sessions engaged as both viewers of, and witnesses to, the lived experiences of veteran peers. This was a silent but effective way to demonstrate that there were other veterans on this same path to healing. Adding an art gallery space that was embedded in the community provided opportunities for veterans to connect to a larger audience through public display of their artwork. Gallery exhibits helped to bridge gaps in understanding and empathy between veterans and civilians by engaging civilians in viewing, witnessing, and learning about veterans lived experiences through their participation as gallery visitors. The range of connections fostered—with the studio, the art itself, and those who viewed the art—helped to reduce the isolation experienced by many veterans during transition.

    Artmaking during open studio sessions among veteran peers was described by the veterans researchers as a psychologically safe way to connect with others. One veteran described, "I've never had a safe place before ... It's safe to share these things here because we all illustrate them" (DeLucia, 2015, p. 49) Noticing the commonalities that were evident between his artwork and the artwork of veteran peers encouraged a sense of emotional safety for this veteran, helping him to open up and receive support from other participating veterans. Attending to the needs of relationships through open communication helped to form healthy, meaningful connections. It also helped to repair previously strained relationships. Veteran artwork served as a voice in these conversations to help significant others understand what the veteran was going through. As one veteran described, "It gives me a chance to let people know what is going on with me" (DeLucia, 2015, p. 50).

    A similar process and benefits occurred as veterans created and prepared their artwork for gallery exhibits. One veteran described his art show experience by saying, "I shared things I've never told anyone. They are still there in my head, but the weight is not there anymore" (DeLucia, 2015, appendix D). He experienced several viewers who attended the exhibit become emotionally moved by his art expressions and the messages communicated through his images about his pain, suffering, and healing. As the veteran researcher discussed this experience, another veteran on the research team shared his experience, and another veteran on the research team shared his own impressions of the exhibit: "You shared something through your art that was extremely personal, and I connected with you on it because we shared similar experiences. I wanted to thank you because your art expression made me realize I could own it too and share it with my therapist. Because of you I am better" (DeLucia, 2015, p. 50). This exchange illustrates a powerful example of how the art show connected veteran and viewer, leaving both positively transformed by the process.

3. **Art therapy draws out strengths.** Veteran researchers described how they developed a sense of mastery over the materials and created artwork they felt was "good." This experience was identified as "a self-esteem builder" that facilitated a sense of accomplishment and bolstered self-efficacy (Franklin, 1992; Kaimal & Ray, 2017). Engaging in art therapy elicited the personal strengths of veterans and helped them reconnect with a healthy, creative, and capable sense of self. In other words, art therapy treated dysfunction by providing opportunities to function (Moon, 2008). And a capable sense of self is needed when engaging with others in community.

4. **Art therapy cultivates a sense of purpose.** Several of the veteran researchers identified two major struggles with transition: reconstructing their identity and reestablishing a sense of purpose. These struggles were related to immediate concerns they expressed about feeling productive. They described how engaging in artmaking helped them to rediscover their innate ability to be creative. In turn, creativity helped them to look at problems and challenges they had identified in new ways and inspired new ideas and solutions. Making art also promoted a sense of freedom and accomplishment as they experimented, learned, and brought their projects to fruition. Completing a project was a satisfying achievement; it helped to build self-esteem, and inspired veterans to consider new alternatives to life challenges. A sense of purpose helps to anchor feelings of belonging.

Conclusion

The community-based approach to art therapy developed and evaluated by and with this local veteran community highlights how studio and gallery components to an art therapy program can provide therapeutic benefits that extend beyond the scope of the individual art therapy session. In many ways they serve to reestablish a sense of care, connection and belonging. Nonclinical approaches to art therapy also help to reduce stigma and facilitate engagement, providing both a bridge into therapy and a transition back into community. Considering how to involve communities served in participatory approaches to program development and evaluation can help to address divides based on lack of understanding or awareness, and orient services around the needs and concerns of the community served. Art therapists are uniquely situated to support community-based and participatory approaches through the range of engagement opportunities the arts provide.

References

Allen, P. B. (1995). Coyote comes in from the cold: The evolution of the open studio concept. *Art Therapy*, *12*(3), 161–166. https://doi.org/10.1080/07421656.1995 .10759153

Caplin, D., & Lewis, K. K. (2011). Coming home: Examining the homecoming experiences of young veterans. In D. C. Kelly, S. Howe-Barksdale, & D. Gitelson (Eds.), *Treating young veterans: Promoting resilience through practice and advocacy* (pp. 101–124). Springer.

DeLucia, J. M., & Kennedy, B. (2021). A veteran-focused art therapy program: Co-Research to strengthen art therapy effectiveness. *International Journal of Art Therapy*, *26*(1–2), 8–16. https://doi.org/10.1080/17454832.2021.1889007

DeLucia, J. M. (2015). *Creating home in an art therapy program for transitioning veterans*. Unpublished doctoral dissertation. Mount Mary University.

DeLucia, J. M. (2016). Art therapy services to support veterans' transition to civilian life: The studio and the gallery. *Art Therapy*, *33*(1), 4–12. https://doi.org/10.1080 /07421656.2016.1127113

Fenner, P. (2012). What do we see? Extending understanding of visual experience in the art therapy encounter. *Art Therapy*, *29*(1), 11–18. https://doi.org/10.1080/07421656 .2012.648075

Franklin, M. (1992). Art therapy and self-esteem. *Art Therapy*, *9*(2), 78–84. https://doi .org/10.1080/07421656.1992.10758941

Furukawa, T. (1997). Sojourner adjustment: Mental health of international students after one year's foreign sojourn and its psychosocial correlates. *Journal of Nervous and Mental Disease*, *185*(4), 263–268. https://doi.org/10.1097/00005053-199704000-00007

Henley, D. (1995). A consideration of the studio as a therapeutic intervention. *Art Therapy*, *12*(3), 188–190. https://doi.org/10.1080/07421656.1995.10759158

Howells, V., & Zelnik, T. (2009). Making art: A qualitative study of personal and group transformation on a community arts studio. *Psychiatric Rehabilitation Journal*, *33*(3), 215–222. https://doi-org.libezproxy2.syr.edu/10.2975/32.3.2009.215.222

Kaimal, G., & Ray, K. (2017). Free art-making in an art therapy open studio: Changes in affect and self-efficacy. *Arts and Health*, *9*(2), 154–166. https://doi-org.libezproxy2 .syr.edu/10.1080/17533015.2016.1217248

Larson, G. E., & Norman, S. B. (2014). Prospective prediction of functional difficulties among recently separated veterans. *Journal of Rehabilitation Research and Development*, *51*(3), 415–428. http://dx.doi.org.libezproxy2.syr.edu/10.1682/JRRD .2013.06.0135

Luzzatto, P. (1997). Short-term art therapy on the acute psychiatric ward: The open session as a psychodynamic development of the studio-based approach. *Inscape: Journal of the British Art Therapy Association*, *2*(1), 2–10. https://doi.org/10.1080 /17454839708413038

McNiff, S. (1988). *Fundamentals of art therapy*. Charles C Thomas.

McNiff, S. (1995). Keeping the studio. *Art Therapy*, *12*(3), 179–183. https://doi.org/10 .1080/07421656.1995.10759156

Moon, B. L. (2008). *Introduction to art therapy: Faith in the product* (2nd ed.). Charles C Thomas.

Moon, B. L. (2010). *Art-based group therapy: Theory and practice*. Charles C Thomas.

Riley, S. (2001). *Group process made visible: Group art therapy*. Brunner-Routledge.
Rubin, J. A. (2005). *Artful therapy*. Wiley.
Sayer, N. A., Noorbaloochi, S., Fraizer, P., Carlson, K., Gravely, A., & Murdoch, M. (2010). Reintegration problems and treatment interests among Iraq and Afghanistan combat veterans receiving VA medical care. *Psychiatry Services, 61*(6), 589–597. https://doi.org/10.1176/ps.2010.61.6.589
Waller, D. (1993). *Group interactive art therapy: Its use in training and treatment*. Routledge.

The Colour Palette

Thahmina Begum

> I knew if I walked into a room with a group of people of color and asked them to talk about racism, there would be silence. The project has reinforced my reasons to become an art therapist and the transformative powers of community art making. I have learned that art therapy is unique, effective, and holds the ability to explore global, social, and political issues that affect everyday lives of individuals and communities.

In 2021, when the world was in a mist of a global pandemic, the question of inequality came to the forefront. However, living in times of great polarized political and social change, the pandemic evoked a great deal of varying issues surrounding poverty, race, displacement of people, and gender. As a British Bangladeshi woman born, educated, and working in the UK, the questions around racism and racial trauma resurfaced for me. I directly feel the impacts of the Black Lives Matter movement, the resulting protests, and the disproportionate effects of COVID-19 Bangladeshi have faced during the pandemic.

Growing up as a child, I knew when somebody looked at me in a strange way or treated me differently but I could not articulate or understand that this was racism. My best friends throughout school were white females, yet there was always a group of people at school that would make me feel different/like I did not belong there. Whether it was saying I had "chip-pan greasy hair," smelled of curry, or I was "a chocolate ice cream," these comments stay vivid and alive in my memory. Trauma is defined as any experience that causes the child unbearable psychic pain or anxiety. For an experience to be unbearable means that it overwhelms the usual defense measures (Kalsched, 1996). This would explain why these hurtful comments have remained in my conscious and unconscious mind, held in my body. As I unlock and reflect on some of my childhood experiences, I now understand them to be experiences of racism.

Having worked for over 20 years in community settings, I have seen first-hand the pain, destruction, and impact of racial trauma on an individual's health; often because the racism is normalized in society "the traumatic stress remains invisible" (Davids, 2009, p. 733 in Tummala-Narra, 2020). Black Asian Minority Ethnic people have died in greater numbers in the pandemic (Highfield, 2020 in Eastwood, 2021) and in the recent Marmot Review (2020) exploring health inequalities in England, Marmot writes that BAME communities have higher mortality risks, due to "longstanding inequalities and structural racism" (p. 19).

Armed with my personal knowledge and experience as well as the theoretical research I did in my art therapy training, I set out to do a community research project where I wasn't just talking and where I created a place for people to share, discuss, reflect, and heal both individually and collectively. Funded through Tetley Art Gallery (Leeds), through their PANIC Bursary Programme, "The Colour Palette" was born.

My project explored the contentious, complex, and personal issue of racial trauma through nine community Creative Laboratories with three different Bangladeshi generational groups. My main question would be: How can art aid healing from racial trauma? My aim with the groups was to define and explore racial trauma, uncover the effects of racial trauma, and work out whether it is "real" trauma. Further goals included the participants coming to understand racial microaggressions and how traumatic stress can affect someone both psychologically and neurologically.

The three groups included young people (aged 12–22 years old), adults (24–45 years old), and older women (55–80 years old). The sessions took place over two sites: Tetley Gallery for the first session, where I focused on the large group artmaking together. The large room in Tetley allowed messy play and artmaking. The remaining sessions took place at a local community center where the participants lived. All three sessions were organized into making, reflecting, and then discussing. I took a Dictaphone to the sessions to record oral stories, comments, and observations through the sessions. As I was leading and facilitating the sessions, it was important for me to work with a photographer who would not only take good quality photographs but also understand the storytelling behind the project. I worked with a wonderful and super-talented lady called Marina. Marina was originally from Armenia; having known Marina for several years I also knew she had suffered racial discrimination. It was important for me to have a person of color as the photographer; I wanted someone who understood, cared about this topic, and, above all, immersed themselves into the sessions as opposed to being an observer. Marina did this seamlessly, like a chameleon, each session instantly gaining the trust of the participants.

Young People

For the first session I set up the large white-walled room with an array of art materials on each table. Materials included paints, inks, chalk, pastels, collage, and clay. I prepared one table with a large white sheet of paper and an outline of a person. I observed that the young people walked into this new space with looks of exactment and anticipation. I directed everyone around the table with the white sheet of paper. Explaining the project and introducing Marina, I quickly moved on to ask them the question: What does racism look, feel, hear, smell, feel like? Working as a group, I asked them to fill in the outline of this body.

The young people looked around at each other, reluctant to start, then one young person started talking of an incident at school. It almost felt like this disclosure was an invitation that gave permission to the other young people to vocalize incidents that had happened to them. As they were talking, they were making, messing, and experimenting with the art materials. I could see their unconscious minds were bringing up many images of the past, mostly about incidents that had happened at school with teachers. The anger, frustration, and complete helplessness on the young people's faces was sad to see. In so many of the incidents the young people reportedly asked for help, justice, yet nothing was done.

One of the most powerful images for me in this session was a polystyrene egg repeatedly painted by participant 6. Firstly, she painted one of them black, then went to the toilets and washed it off. She then took another egg and painted it peach and then washed it off in the toilets. When I asked her about this, she said we are all like eggs, our skins may be different colors on the outside but inside, just like there is a yolk, we all have the same-colored heart. It was so powerful, and, in that moment, I knew the power of artmaking was real and absolute magic. Many of the young people spoke of how they had never had an opportunity to talk about this issue anywhere and especially not at home, as most family members think you must get over it or just don't understand.

Adults

The adult group was very different from the young people group. As soon as we started the group making, every single participant had so much to say, story after story, incident after incident. Many participants reflected on similar incidents that had happened to them, again not having had an opportunity to talk about how they felt in the body when racism happened. When I explained about how the stress of racism affects our bodies, it was like a "light bulb" moment for the participants. I could see around the room faces agreeing, understanding, and contemplating. One participant commented, "Now I understand why I felt angry for days and this feeling just wouldn't go away." The first session with this group felt heavy for me; there was a great deal to hold, facilitating so many stories. I felt like I had opened a can of worms, and they were just slithering everywhere! So many violent, emotional, verbal, subtle incidents of racism, from being at school, growing up, and workplace environments.

In the second session I wanted to concentrate on the participants' emotions. I chose to provide only black charcoal and white paper on the table. I asked the participants to draw their emotions from one of the racist incidents they had described the previous session. The atmosphere in the room went silent; I could see the focus on the participants' faces. I asked if they would like to share and talk about their images with the group. One participant spoke about how she didn't know what she was doing but then suddenly, all this stuff came out! For me this highlighted the transformative power of artmaking.

The most powerful session with this group was the final session, when I asked them to reflect on the two sessions and then write a letter to their racist. I was expecting reluctance, but all the participants eagerly started writing. I could see the individual and collective growth in them. The mixed emotions written all over the participants faces while writing, painted a thousand words! Once finished, I asked if each participant would like to read their letter to the rest of the group. With each letter, there is so much hurt, sadness, and pain in the stories and experiences of racism. One participant said, "It felt like therapy!" Others spoke about how much better they felt after reading their letter, as if they had taken power back from their perpetrators. They spoke the golden words: art feels like therapy!

Older People

Out of all the groups, this was honestly my most difficult. Immediately the older participants had a look of mistrust about myself, and, especially Marina. One participant quite aggressively said, "Tell her to stop taking my picture!" I knew instantly the first group activity wouldn't work. Very quickly I put chairs in a circle and started a conversation around racism in their mother tongue language and dialect Sylheti. This quickly built trust and conversation around the trauma of moving to a new country and not being allowed to talk about the issue of racism as these acts were completely normalized in the 1970/80s. They spoke about how they had to "put up and shut up!" Many participants had held on to this racial trauma for 40 or 50 years. They were scared to talk about it in case they got into trouble or made trouble for their families. In some cases, they were told they would get arrested! It was amazing how the participants could remember the exact time, location, and their emotions of the incidents that had happened, even though it was decades ago.

Conclusion

When I set out to deliver the Colour Palette project, my principal aim was to explore how art can heal racial trauma and the effectiveness of community artmaking in healing. I knew if I walked into a room with a group of people of color and asked them to talk about racism, there would be silence. The project has reinforced my reasons for becoming an art therapist and the transformative powers of community artmaking. I have learned that art therapy is unique, effective, and holds the ability to explore global, social, and political issues that affect the everyday lives of individuals and communities.

The Colour Palette project has been extremely successful due to many factors. Having a safe space in which to explore highly sensitive and emotional stories has invited collective voice and expression. The creative labs gave participants tools for imagination and expression and invited them to claim their right to exist as a Bangladeshi person in a white person's world. The artwork provided visual resonance to the participants' experiences, and a way to externalize internalized racism. This resonance helped to deepen trust among the participants quickly through speaking about their experiences. The support from the Tetley team and Marina allowed autonomy and enabled me to develop this project. Community art therapy invited individuals to collectively identify racist experiences, process their emotions and feelings related to racism, and reclaim their power. Art therapy truly makes a difference to people's lives.

References

Eastwood, C. (2021). White privilege and art therapy in the UK: Are we doing the work? *International Journal of Art Therapy* [Online]. Available https://doi.org/10.1080/17454832.2020.1856159

Kalshed, D. (1996). *The Inner World of Trauma; Archetypal defences of the personal spirit*. Routledge.

Marmot, M. (2020). *Build back fairer: The COVID-19 marmot review. The pandemic, socioeconomic and health inequalities in England*. Institute of Health Equity.

Tummala-Narra, P. (2020). Racial trauma and dissociated worlds within psychotherapy: A discussion of "racial difference, rupture, and repair: A view from the couch and back". *Psychoanalytic Dialogues*, *30*(6), 732–741. https://doi.org/10.1080/10481885.2020.1829437

In the Hands of Community

Implications of a Liberatory, Systemic View of Practice

Lynn Kapitan

Our focus has never been to train individuals to practice art therapy; rather, art therapy is a liberatory tool in training participants to become capable change agents in their communities. Acutely aware that we all are related to one another, no one is left behind and without full participation in their self-determination. In such a context, if you have something of value, you must share it; you must open your hands and give it away.

Many years ago, high up in the Andes mountains of Peru, I was traveling along a rutted, winding road that gradually descended into the sacred valley of the Urubamba. There was no moon but, because we were at high altitude and far from any town or even homestead, the sky was teeming with stars, the glorious Milky Way more resplendent than I've ever known. Awestruck, I gazed upon this river of stars reflected in the river of the Urubamba. All at once, in that moment, I grasped a piece of Andean cosmology: how perfectly balanced the upper, and middle, and lower worlds are, and our places within them. The river above is a mirror image of the river below it; that is a mirror of the unseen, deeper river far below our feet; all is interconnected. Each of us, as a living being, is related to every other being, past and present. We are community.

When I reflect on 20 years of community-based art therapy practice, this star-filled image of sacred interconnectivity arises in me, still inspiring everything I think and do. My very understanding of art therapy has changed. I no longer perceive it as a single profession; rather, I have come to know art therapy as an expansive social geography, comprising many communities of practice (Kapitan, 2014; Wenger, 1998), encamped along the sacred river of creative energy we draw on for our work. Each community, near or far, imbues art therapy with its own unique knowledge, practices, resources, and perspectives yet shares a common purpose, which unites us in our diversity. In this polarized time of political, technological, and social upheaval, a systemic view is plainly needed. By itself, art will never be enough; knowledge is not enough. Healing requires relationship and a willingness to work across boundaries of difference, to imagine, as Arundati Roy said, that "another world is not only possible, she is on her way" (2003, p. 75).

I believe in such a world, thanks in large part to my work with Cantera, a Nicaraguan non-governmental health and education organization. Founded in the 1970s by Anabel Torres in the time of dictatorship and enduring through the country's revolution, civil war, economic collapse, and return to authoritarianism, Cantera's vision is explicitly grounded in social justice, toward the achievement of a more equitable and sustainable society that permits the ethical and spiritual fulfillment of all its people. Cantera invests in rural and urban Nicaraguan communities through projects that attend to the needs of children, youth, and families; address disparities; and create small-scale economies aimed at food security, sustainability, and environmental justice. These projects are not meant to fix problems but to build the dreams of the community. The "dream that moves us is the transformation of our reality," explains Torres (as cited in Cantera, n.d.). "We think that it is important to define our dreams for ourselves, our families, and our communities [and] we use them to be the starting point of our projects. We accompany an array of people, regardless of gender, age, beliefs, etc., on this journey toward social transformation."

The Interconnected, Systemic Mindset of Community Art Therapy Practice

I was invited to integrate community-based art therapy into Cantera's model of *popular education*, which refers to education by and for ordinary people in the service of liberation, self-determination, and change (Freire, 1970). Each encounter begins with recognizing and naming the participants' social realities through a questioning, critical analysis. Whatever arises in that process is explored through creative arts practices for finding common ground and for dreaming, planning, and analyzing collective actions. The goal is not therapy but transformation on a community and societal scale. Women, youth, elders, farmers, folk healers, educators, and others who are recognized by their communities as natural leaders participate in focused trainings that strengthen identity, leadership, self-efficacy, and voice. Building this capacity in individuals effects an impact on their families and, in turn, their community and society.

It is nearly impossible to convey the powerful impact this practice has had on my own identity and knowledge over the years. Most striking to me is how it has shifted my mental model, especially in light of my US-based professional training and cultural conditioning. Where I once saw individuals in need, I now see those individuals in relation to complex, interconnected social networks of support and help. In the hands of a community, art therapy is not simply a site of practice comprising groups or individual clients; rather, the "client" is the entire community (Kapitan et al., 2011). This shift in thinking reveals the interconnectedness of micro and macro realities. For example, from neuroscience we know that to develop healthy brain circuitry, an individual needs an abundance of healthy experiences. Likewise, on the community scale of practice, art therapy can facilitate healthy social circuitry, which fortifies the community's immune system to resist the toxins of oppression and other social ills.

What distinguishes community practice from group art therapy, in my experience, is that it incorporates *a systemic vision of reality* that recognizes the interconnectedness of all life elements: the individual and the collective self; the local and the global; the economic and the cultural; the material and spiritual worlds, and more. Any single change initiates a process of change in the entire system (Cantera, n.d.). While healing the body-mind may be the focus of individual art therapy, community art therapy is equally committed to healthy, free, and creative minds in a free, dynamic, and just social body, as Martín-Baró (1996) asserted. Community is a way of thinking, as well as a therapeutic goal, the process or means by which that goal is achieved, and the co-creator of that process.

Surrendering to the Empowered Community

When the community—and not art therapy—is the central force of change, the art therapist must be elastic enough to shift and be transformed as well (Kapitan,

2014). This has meant allowing the community to use me as they would an art material (Kapitan et al., 2011), to shape and be shaped in whatever direction we require. As an "art material," I am regarded as a precious resource needed "to make the community's dreams come true" (Cantera, n.d.); that is, to be maximally malleable, responsive, and made suitable for cultural expression, as well as collectively shared so that everyone in the entire community benefits. Coming from an individualistic culture, this surrender to the collective once felt irritating (and even alarming) to me. However, I now understand that by ceding power and control, the benefits of art therapy can move through community support networks while ensuring culturally logical uses of my knowledge, skills, ideas, and resources.

Evidence and implications of the dynamics between the community and myself as the art therapist can be found in the evolution of change over time. When I started working in Nicaragua, there were no art materials. Political and economic repression over the course of generations had severed people from their own folk traditions and artistic inheritance. But after only a few years, a distinctly Nicaraguan form of art therapy began to emerge throughout the country. I attribute this change not solely to the liberating power of art but to the "multiplier effect" of community empowerment: to carry out their collective projects, every participant who attends one of Cantera's trainings commits to returning to their community to teach others what they have learned, sharing their knowledge with as many people as possible.

From a dominant cultural perspective, this free sharing of art therapy raises discomfort, often framed in ethical terms: If ordinary people are taught art therapy and then teach it to others, doesn't that put people at risk for incompetent care? What of the danger of untrained professionals practicing on an unsuspecting public? But my own experience tells me that this is not what is happening here. In the case of Cantera, comprehensive program evaluation research (Kapitan et al., 2011) found no lack of understanding among a wide spectrum of participants regarding the ethical boundaries of art therapy practice. In fact, the notion that participants might use their training to practice as a professional art therapist was regarded as absurd. To make sense of this finding, we must put aside a culture-bound assumption that the ethical rules we have been taught are universal, or worse, that just because one has not perceived an alternative set of rules operating in a given situation does not mean no such rules exist.

A Community Ethics of Care

A closer look reveals several ethical structures that protect and support care, all of which are grounded in relationship and reciprocal obligations and accountability. Community art therapy in Nicaragua, as facilitated by Cantera and my role within it, rests on deeply held cultural values of respect, caring, equitable treatment of one another, and, more specifically, the social justice principles of popular education (Freire, 1970). A relational ethics of responsibility arises from a holistic approach to reality, attentive to the balance of personal and communal, body and spirit, and "the dreams and realities we seek to transform" (Cantera, n.d.). In low-income countries where there is scant access to higher education, trained professionals, and mental health care, it would be irresponsible and unethical to *not* share beneficial art therapy practices wherever possible.

The practice of *task sharing* can shed light on the community dissemination of art therapy that is occurring in low-income countries such as Nicaragua. Defined as the strategic redistribution of certain tasks, from highly trained health care professionals to lay people or those with shorter training or fewer qualifications (Orkin et al., 2021), task sharing is being used across the globe to address severe disparities between mental health needs and access to professional care. Research has found that task sharing is effective: the acceptance and use of helpful interventions increase when they are delivered by trustworthy community members, as they are more likely than professionals to share the community's local cultural, linguistic, and social backgrounds (Orkin et al., 2021). A systemic mindset helps the art therapist task share in the direction of community needs. In my case, by placing basic psychosocial art therapy techniques in the hands of local Nicaraguan community members, I am freed to focus higher-level expertise on training, supervision, and case consultation, all of which multiply benefits further. To monitor community applications of new knowledge, Cantera's fieldwork teams visit between trainings to help sustain their projects and, during these visits, provide supervision, personal support, and ethical guidance.

In community-based art therapy, in-depth knowledge of the community within all its sociocultural contexts is vital; the therapist's cultural humility is founded on it. I recall a participant in Nicaragua who experienced community art therapy as "a light that walks with us and accompanies our thoughts, feelings, and actions, opening our hearts as well as our minds" while strengthening interior life "as a counter-force to society's negative forces" (Kapitan et al., 2011, p. 71). Our focus has never been to train individuals to practice art therapy; rather, art therapy is a liberatory tool in training participants to become capable change agents in their communities. Acutely aware that we all are related to one another, no one is left behind and without full participation in their self-determination. In such a context, if you have something of value, you must share it; you must open your hands and give it away.

Community Resilience and Beauty to Counteract Oppression and Fear

Community art therapy has made me porous, having taught me to turn toward suffering and bring my full presence to it, allow it to affect me, to matter to me, to alter my course (Watkins, 2015). When a horrific political conflict took hold of Nicaragua in 2018, leaving hundreds of people dead and thousands imprisoned or exiled, I became newly conscious of how vital art therapy was to the community in the face of oppression. Although the crisis had cut them off from Cantera's support, several communities mobilized to protect each other from the violence and turned to their art therapy knowledge to strategize their survival. Six months later, gathering at a Cantera retreat at our first opportunity, I witnessed these cherished companions of mine, my heart catching in my throat. In the darkened room, small groups of all ages and backgrounds were seated on the floor around watercolors and cups of water. Together we silently painted by candlelight, which symbolized finding hope in the darkness, lighted by the spirit of community that nourished and drew us together, despite the continuing danger. We acknowledged the fear and suffering, but also affirmed strengths, beauty, and resilience. Caring in community, I believe, is the only way we will heal our broken world.

In the three years since that time, the global pandemic has descended upon us all, further straining our ability to find connection with one another. And, in my own home community, a terrible struggle persists against police brutality, political repression, and systemic racism. On the night I smelled the smoke of burning buildings, I suddenly remembered painting by candlelight in Nicaragua. Holding the image in mind, I felt the warmth and resolve of the resilient community, now sustaining me. Everything is connected. What is above is below, what is there is also here. We cannot escape the differing locations we find ourselves in. But we can listen closely and share the diversity and commonality of our experiences and commit to multiplying the impacts of this work.

All over the world, among the many stories and images that arise in art therapy, are those seeking release from oppression. When practiced in community, people are not just using art to collectively make things; they are opening themselves to a larger whole of which they are a part. They create art out of living memories to celebrate or to shed new light on shared events. They touch one another through story, dance, and rituals; they practice seeing and feeling and participating in the world around them. They dissolve the dreadful power of fear and despair that otherwise keeps us isolated and separate. In community-based art therapy we look outward as well as inward. We engage in a collective dream life where hopes and ideas, histories, current realities, and new ways of going forward are realized.

References

Cantera. (n.d.). Letter from our director. http://canteranicaragua.org/en/who-are-we/a
    -letter-from-our-director/

Freire, P. (1970). *Pedagogy of the oppressed*. Plenum Press.

Kapitan, L. (2014). Re: Invention and realignments of art therapy. *Art Therapy Online*,
    5(1). https://doi.org/10.25602/GOLD.atol.v5i1.328

Kapitan, L., Litell, M., & Torres, A. (2011). Creative art therapy in a community's participatory research and social transformation. *Art Therapy: Journal of the American Art Therapy Association, 28*(2), 64–73. https://doi.org/10.1080/07421656.2011.578238

Martín-Baró, I. (1996). *Writings for a liberation psychology* (A. Aron, S. Corne, & E. G. Mischler, eds.). Harvard University Press.

Martiniuk, A., Salamanca-Buentello, F., & Upshur, R. (2021). Conceptual framework for task shifting and task sharing: An international Delphi study. *Human Resources for Health, 19*(61). https://doi.org/10.1186/s12960-021-00605-z

Orkin, A., Rao, S., Venugopal, J., Kithulegoda, N., Wegier, P., Ritchie, S., VanderBurgh, D., Martiniuk, A., Salamanca-Buentello, F., & Upshur, R. (2021). Conceptual framework for task shifting and task sharing: An international Delphi study. *Human Resources for Health, 19*(61), 1–8. https://doi.org/10.1186/s12960-021-00605-z

Roy, A. (2003). *War talk*. South End Press.

Watkins, M. (2015). Psychosocial accompaniment. *Journal of Social and Political Psychology, 3*(1), 324–342. https://doi.org/10.5964/jspp.v3i1.103

Wenger, E. (1998). *Communities of practice: Learning, meaning, and identity*. Cambridge University Press.

Learning Through Loss

Fostering Community Connections for Adjudicated Adolescents

Laura Swift

What followed was a whirlwind of months comprised of extensive conversations, planning, creating, and compromising, which culminated in a wildly successful grand opening followed by a devastatingly premature termination of the program. The lessons I learned from this experience ultimately allowed me to become a better art therapist as they helped me to narrow my clinical focus, provided perspective, and showed me the power of connection in the therapeutic relationship. I have utilized the lessons learned through the difficult loss of this program to create more sustainable community-based projects.

In early 2015, I was employed by a large nonprofit in Milwaukee, Wisconsin known for their work with youth involved in the juvenile justice system. Within the agency, I was the only art therapist working in a residential treatment program established as an alternative to circumvent the Department of Corrections. Recognizing the potential of art as a powerful resource, the agency invited me to create an arts-based program in a nearby suburb. The original intention of the program was to bring a positive light to the mission of the agency, essentially rebranding the organization by utilizing art to connect to the community in a visible way. I was beyond ecstatic for this opportunity. Though early on in my conversations with the agency I was aware that leadership's vision may be short-sighted, I was confident that I could create a program that aligned their interests with the needs of my clients as well as the needs of the community. What followed was a whirlwind of months comprising extensive conversations, planning, creating, and compromising, which culminated in a wildly success-ful grand opening followed by a devastatingly premature termination of the program. The lessons I learned from this experience ultimately allowed me to become a better art therapist as they helped me to narrow my clinical focus, provided perspective, and showed me the power of connection in the therapeutic relationship. I have utilized the lessons learned through the difficult loss of this program to create more sustainable community-based projects. I have also had the privilege of including youth from the failed program in additional commu-nity projects as they expressed interest, highlighting the need and the power of connection and belonging.

As planning began, I recruited a skilled colleague, fellow art therapist Stephanie Gibart, as a partner in this process. Stephanie was working in the school-based programming of the agency and was equally enthralled by the potential of this opportunity. We had both observed shortcomings within the agency, most notably the absence of a continuation of care after youth returned home from treatment or incarceration. Based on this limitation, the focus of our proposal was to provide a supportive bridge, helping youth to reintegrate into the community by offering opportunities to participate in arts-based programming outside of the traditional walls of the organization. An additional employee, Anna Jarecki Cure, was provided by the agency as a graphic designer and com-munity liaison to round out our team. Her enthusiasm and support helped to create a program that was both visible and accessible through her connections to the neighborhood and other artists, the creation and distribution of brochures, and her seemingly endless energetic support of the mission. Our primary goal was to provide a safe environment for the agency's youth to interact with non-adjudicated youth and members of the community without the stigma of their judicial involvement, mental health needs, or socioeconomic status. Essentially, we wanted this program to provide them opportunities to be kids, while simulta-neously offering them the chance to reframe their perceptions of self. We inter-viewed neighbors, leaders, and staff in the organization, and, most importantly, we questioned the youth involved throughout our process.

What resulted was the YES, ETC collective, building from the agency's existing job readiness program (Youth Employment Services) to include Empowerment Through Creativity. The program included a reciprocal process, where artists from the community would donate time, teaching their craft to groups of youth (both from the agency and the community) in exchange for the opportunity to display their art in the available gallery space. Youth were then invited to exhibit their art alongside that of the professional artists, furthering the opportunity for youth to shift their perspectives of self to include that of being artists.

Early in planning, it seemed that the agency was vocal about their needs, concerns, and goals for the program. The agency leaders were looking to change perceptions of the organization through positive community work and highlighting the existence of art therapists on staff in several programs. Leadership also instructed us to create a signature bracelet that was sold to raise funds for the program. Several difficult conversations occurred around the ethical concerns that Stephanie and I brought forth. We strongly advocated for youth to be reimbursed for their work. As the youth were included in the planning, they requested not only ways to earn money but also ways to earn community service hours and means to pay back their court fees. We structured the program to include opportunities for fundraising, where the youth would create directive-based art with positive messages and receive community service hours in exchange for their time. The completed artwork was sold to raise funds for the program. Stephanie and I strongly felt that if youth chose to sell personal art that was created independently, they should receive the funds, once the cost of materials was recouped by the agency. We proposed putting structures in place to first forward money earned toward paying any outstanding restitution. However, this disagreement over ethics was never resolved with the leadership in the agency, as they did not want youth to receive any monetary compensation for their participation. Eventually, this conflict became one of the reasons that the program was dismantled by the agency.

Throughout the planning process, we enlisted the help of youth involved to advocate for themselves and provide feedback based on their needs, rather than attempting to assign needs to them. Youth identified one primary need that we felt was simple: a space where they could relax and feel like kids, outside of mental health needs or criminogenic behavior. Many of the youth talked about grieving the loss of childhood and a "normal" high school experience. Though many of us who had stereotypically "normal" high school involvement may question the allure, my colleagues and I recognized the loss felt by the kids. In my experience, adjudicated youth tend to feel disempowered and lack control due to reliance on "the system" to determine their progress and readiness to transition home. The highly structured nature of residential treatment leaves little to no room for decision-making and can leave youth going through the motions of progress without authentically making their own choices along the way. Due to this dynamic, my colleagues and I intentionally incorporated choice into every level of this program. Youth were able to choose whether they participated and actively defined their level of participation. They chose the theme of each gallery show, whether they made art collectively or independently, what materials they used, and whether they wanted to display or sell their finished product. Stephanie and I believed that giving youth opportunities to make decisions, even small creative decisions, could help to build self-esteem, self-efficacy, and improve the likelihood of making positive choices outside of peer influence. We wanted to provide opportunities for the youth in the system to participate in structured play, working collaboratively with each other as well as non-adjudicated youth from the community without differentiation.

The success of this program seemed imminent due to several factors. The low overhead expenses, passionate dedication to the mission, and perceived need for this service were all components that led us to believe that we were creating a sustainable program. There was little to no cost to the organization, as the building where YES, ETC was located was generously donated by a board member. Initially, the location seemed ideal: an old brick building in a quaint downtown village with significant walking traffic and ample parking nearby. Yet, as the program progressed, feedback I received from my clients as well as some of the neighbors started to indicate a mutual uneasiness and hesitance to collaborate. Through the process of introducing ourselves and our mission to the community, we were met with a mix of support and resistance.

Milwaukee is one of the most segregated cities in the country, in a state that leads the country in the incarceration of black males (Nellis et al., 2021). Meanwhile, its suburban towns are largely composed of white people. Consequently, the predominately white population of the small suburban town and the Black and Brown kids who comprised the majority of our program were brought together in a way that seemed to be regarded as uncommon in this socio-cultural region. Though we encountered many people who were excited and enthusiastically supportive of our mission, there seemed to be just as many who were guarded and openly resistant to inviting our clients into *their* community. Some neighbors were supportive and willing to donate time, money, and fundraising efforts. Other neighbors were outwardly negative and contributed an element of "not in my back yard" as we attempted to passionately explain our mission. Also, despite our best efforts to protect the anonymity of the youth and their involvement in the juvenile justice system, we found that the agency's reputation superseded our efforts in some cases. Many neighbors expressed fear about bringing adjudicated youth to their town and expressed concern about crime rates rising as a result. Yet, we soon became very aware that our presence as three white women advocating for our clients in the community appeared to help to ease the comfort level in some individuals.

Meanwhile, most of the youth in our program explicitly felt their otherness in this predominantly white suburb. Like some of the neighbors expressing fear and the perceived loss of a sense of safety, in my conversations with my clients I quickly discovered that they also did not feel safe in this neighborhood. They told me that they felt unwanted and ostracized. As I walked down the street with several 15-year-old boys, I experienced the energy shift around me. I felt the hard looks and long stares. Noticing my clients holding a strong posture and hypervigilant observation, I felt them cling closely to me for safety. I observed the narrow, assessing looks from some neighbors, their glances so different than when I walked down this same street alone.

Despite these discrepancies, my fellow organizers and I felt fueled and motivated by the more positive and supportive conversations. The program that we worked to create aimed to balance reciprocity, constantly assessing the needs of the youth, the agency, and the community.

The grand opening was largely a success. We had invited artists from the community as well as youth to create art based on the theme of "empowerment." We worked with the youth to understand and define what empowerment meant to them, and transform their pieces into gallery-ready art. All the professional artists who contributed pieces had agreed to teach classes to youths in future months. The event was attended by youth, agency staff members, the youth's families, members of the court system including judges and attorneys, the professional artists and their own families, as well as curious foot traffic that wandered in. We observed proud kids pointing out and explaining their pieces to family members and strangers. We witnessed family photos posted in front of the gallery walls, as mothers beamed with pride. Art became a tangible connective conduit between youth and the community, providing a positive shift in their sense of self as well as in the community's perception. Several youth sold paintings at the grand opening, including one youth who, to his amazement, sold his painting on the street to a passerby. Once material costs were recovered, the remaining profit was reserved for the young people. Professional artists were also offered the opportunity to donate some or all of their profits back into the program.

We were riding high on the excitement and success of this initial gallery opening, but immediately began to focus on the next month's theme. We had received a lot of donated supplies, including hundreds of white 4 × 4 tiles, and sat brainstorming potential uses for the material. One youth suggested that they write the names of each person who had died from gun violence that year on the tiles to create a wall installation in the gallery. From that conversation, the youth chose the theme of stopping the violence in Milwaukee for the next show, as this had been a significantly deadly year in our city. As we were working on the tiles, a staff member came into the art room, picked up a tile tenderly, and asked "Why is my cousin's name on this?" When a young person explained the process, the staff member asked whether he could help and got to work carving the names of several other people's lost loved ones into other tiles. The reciprocal process continued in ways that we could not have foreseen.

Unfortunately, weeks into preparing for our next show and only two months after our grand opening I was brought into the office of the CEO and told that the community space would be shut down, effective immediately. The reason provided for the cut was that it "didn't bring in enough money," because we had lost out on a grant opportunity. Despite arguments for additional funding, other grants, and again the low overhead costs, the program was closed, and I was left answering to the youth who had become invested in the program. We were all heartbroken and angry. We took some time to nurse our wounds, but ultimately realized that we couldn't create a sustainable program within an agency that didn't see the value of what we had done. The lessons I learned from this experience and loss, however, have been sustainable in many ways that allowed me to shift my perspective from that of failure to that of a powerful learning experience that made me a better clinician and human.

I discovered that having a strong partner in this process not only helped to ease the burden, but also provided endless inspiration. Stephanie and I spent many late nights brainstorming creative and practical solutions to problems, imagining best- and worst-case scenarios in the name of safety and ethics, outlining goals and dreaming as big as we could. There may have been a lot of wine and giggles, but ultimately, we were passionately focused on working within the limits of the agency to provide the most effective and impactful opportunities for our clients.

I also learned that location is as important, if not more important, than the mission of a program. If individuals can't get to services or don't feel safe in the neighborhood in which the resources are located, clients are not being served. Many of the youth involved shared that they enjoyed the program but were unsure whether they would continue to attend after returning home because of the inaccessibility and perceived lack of safety of the neighborhood. In my work since this experience, I have ensured that I am working in neighborhoods that are accessible to my clients and that they are surrounded by people who look like them. This often means that I am the only white woman in a space. This shift in my practice has helped me to learn some humbling lessons, which I have been able to take into my daily work to become a more culturally competent and empathic clinician.

This experience also helped me to learn ways to better determine the needs of the community through ongoing conversations with the community. Rather than assuming or assigning needs without having the same lived experience, I worked to establish rapport and safety to create an environment where my clients and the community in which I was working felt comfortable enough to express their honest opinions and needs.

On a personal level, I learned that I am passionate about finding and filling gaps in services to help youth connect. This process ignited my passion for community-based art therapy and led to some of the most fulfilling moments of my career. In the years following this project, I joined Bloom, a community-based art therapy practice on the south side of Milwaukee. To make use of some of the lessons I learned, I connected with my friend, Dr. Chuck Holloway, who owns a youth-focused agency on the north side of Milwaukee. We worked out a barter where I ran a weekly art therapy group for youth in exchange for an office to work out of the rest of the week. The location was far more accessible for my clients. An additional benefit of this arrangement is that the groups were open to the community, and I was able to invite former and current clients to make art alongside other youth and I in a non-directive studio art group. We worked to create several murals to cover the walls of the building and I felt a sense of completion when several of the youth who had been a part of the failed collective not only attended but also contributed to the creation. I was over-joyed to see them pick up paintbrushes as one youth, now a young man, told me: "Look what you got us doing, Ms. Laura. I feel like we're kids again." I felt privileged to witness the joy and amazement in their process as we worked creatively in tandem on something visible and sustainable. It was not lost on me that this experience, as well as our primary goal of kids being able to feel like kids, was made possible by the failed efforts of the first collective. The lessons I learned through the loss made room for new and powerful opportunities.

I began to view my role in this process as a conductor, creating a safe space for people to connect by allowing energy to flow through me and the creative process. Through this lens I created a space in the community where my former clients felt comfortable attending groups with youth and adults who were not involved in the juvenile justice system—a place where they were able to feel like kids again while working alongside, and helping, each other through the creative process.

One program ended, but many more creative paths opened, changing not only the perspectives of the youth and the communities where we operated, but also ours as the creative practitioners. As an art therapist, it feels like a true gift of the profession to be able to witness the organic connection between art and community. Art brought people together who would otherwise not have intersected and inspired change, hope, and connectivity.

References

Nellis, A., Rovner, J., & Porter, N. D. (2021, November 1). *The color of justice: Racial and ethnic disparity in state prisons*. The Sentencing Project. Retrieved January 28, 2022, from https://www.sentencingproject.org/publications/color-of-justice-racial-and-ethnic-disparity-in-state-prisons/

Reflection on Community and School Art Therapy Internships

Dani Moss

In our supervision, we worked on 'the approach' aspect of community art therapy.

Like a pollinator (Moss, 2017), the art therapist transfers their unique skills with the community or system with whom and where they work. Oftentimes it is art therapists in training during their internships who pollinate new landings in the social realm with art therapy, but the conditions must be right to support the interaction. Conditions include site supervision from supervisors who have specific qualifications and agree to complete evaluations and administrative tasks, and opportunities to complete adequate direct client contact hours. Supervisors must also be willing to oversee the unique work of the art therapy intern, even if they are not art therapists themselves. Finding the right conditions can be challenging.

In my role as a graduate art therapy educator and internship coordinator in Western Pennsylvania I help to "find paths" for art therapy. I have helped to forge, foster, and support art therapy internships in a variety of vetted and new settings such as schools, community agencies, private practices, medical systems, community outreach programs, and non-mental health institutions. As an academic art therapy supervisor instructing internship courses, I balance tasks of instructing, grading (Deaver, 2012), and facilitating supervision.

To illustrate some dynamics of internship arrangements in community settings I will share a few case examples. All names are used with permission.

Teen Drop-In Center

Sarah Baker, a participant in the research for the grounded theory and the beehive model of community art therapy presented in this book, completed an art therapy internship in a community setting where she worked with community members to prepare a concept map for a community mural celebrating generations. The setting where she completed her internship was in a partnership of two sister organizations in a neighborhood borough at the perimeter of Pittsburgh, PA, city limits. One was a community outreach teen drop-in center and one was an outpatient therapy practice that took private insurance, private pay, and Medicare. The neighborhood residents had generational ties and the infrastructure and businesses had rich history.

The individual who was qualified per accreditation requirements to provide site supervision worked as a licensed counselor in the private practice portion of the partnership. The site supervisor had not yet supervised anyone in her career and was open to learning about art therapy. Baker obtained most of her clinical direct hours in the teen drop-in center, however. The arrangement strained the site supervisor in that she needed to give up time in the outpatient clinic and spend unpaid time observing the art therapy services in the drop-in center. Additionally, in time, the site supervisor transitioned away from the organization and the sister sites settled on the owner of the outpatient clinic taking on the site supervisory role so that Baker could complete the internship.

The teen drop-in center leaders modeled their community counseling services from a multicultural social justice perspective (Lewis et al., 2010). The culture of "treatment" was vastly different than in the outpatient clinic and the therapists and counselors had a variety of helper training. Baker, a young white woman who moved to the area for graduate training, needed to enter the community and collaborate with colleagues with cultural humility. The site had many interns from related fields, but Baker was the only master's-level art therapy intern, which caused some confusion because of her unique supervisory and direct client contact needs. Inclusion via intake differed in the drop-in center and Baker was challenged with interpreting how theoretical approaches and assessment translated from behind closed outpatient doors in a session where clients received diagnoses into the open gymnasium and community rooms where social and relational issues were the focus.

It is due to the open inclusion criteria of the community drop-in center, however, that Baker was presented with the opportunity to transcend the walls and venture into the surrounding neighborhood. In class, I supported Baker as she shifted her goals of "art therapy." As Baker's academic supervisor, I framed her work in methodologies of arts-based and participatory action research paradigms to help her make sense of what she was doing. My experience as an art therapy researcher gave us theoretical underpinning to support her approaches. The process of obtaining permissions and objectives required time and communication between stakeholders. Baker was part of all communications and steered the scope of any projects that she facilitated so that she was not overwhelmed by meeting her training program learning objectives and defining community art therapy practice.

Art Museum

A second example of a challenging community art therapy internship arrangement took place in a major art museum institution in Pittsburgh, PA. The art therapy intern, Taylor, was able to locate paths in the institution because she was an employee and had a working relationship already established with the director of educational outreach.

When the time came for Taylor to start her master's-level art therapy and counseling internship, arrangement stakeholders came together for a brainstorming and collaborative meeting. I met with Taylor, the museum's education director, and a staff member from human services and payroll. We reviewed the requirements of the internship and discussed how "mental health" or "art therapy" would be defined and provided at the site. The "site" included the museum itself as well as two other preexisting community partners in the outreach program. The arrangement became complex, but all parties verbally committed to supporting a successful internship. Supervision would be provided by a contracted credentialed therapist who would receive a stipend from the museum.

The museum eventually underwent structural changes that complicated and pre-vented a frequency of communications that were needed to support Taylor and compensate the contracted professional art therapist. Taylor and one partnership site could not agree on what "community art therapy" services should look like and did not gain traction to a point where Taylor was collecting any direct hours toward her internship.

Taylor lived near one of the partner organizations and identified as a member of the community. As a young art therapist and woman of color, her stake in her community work was personal and she looked forward to facilitating a "soft entry" into therapy by focusing her work on wellness, psychoeducation, and cre-ative expression. Her familiarity and expectations of her community proved to be both strength and challenge. In campus supervision we deferred to Ottemiller and Awais' (2016) community-based model for art therapists to help Taylor further define how she was engaging and maneuvering in an egalitarian way, yet taking leadership as a facilitator of services with her art therapist skills. As she learned to manage hierarchies, she worked through fears of positioning herself as a "savior." In the community setting it was difficult for her to differentiate predictable therapy relationship dynamics without clearer definition.

The whole group of stakeholders were navigating multiple organizational systems' communications, structures, schedules, and so forth. For example, Taylor needed to communicate with the director of one of the partner sites to find time to be on site and join with the setting but was also answering to the umbrella "site" who hosted the partnership, her site supervisor, and her academic supervi-sor. Each organization and entity had their own professional culture and Taylor needed to adapt her learnings and approach. Taylor was essentially developing programming in three different brick-and-mortar organizations as well as in a neighborhood. The museum's culture was steeply different from those of the community partners. In our supervision we worked on "the approach" aspect of community art therapy, attempting to help Taylor feel secure in her work as she traveled physically and virtually into varying spaces. In some spaces she was a consistent group leader, in others she created pop-up artmaking with the goal of connection and sharing for people who were gathering at locations for resources.

Through our supervision discussions we grouped all organizations as "the community" and framed the community as "the client" to help Taylor man-age the enormity of the work, because I deferred to family systems theory as a frame for joining and Taylor cleverly used metaphor and created a case con-ceptualization using a family systems assessment of the neighborhood where she was working and its "family" members in relation to the metropolitan city at large. Through this assessment, Taylor identified relational needs, economic factors, racial inequities, historical trauma, and through a hermeneutic reflection, articulated embodied expressions of inter- and intrapersonal relationships and medical illness trends. Taylor's assessment helped clarify needs which helped her to prepare art therapy services, yet also created overwhelm and a sense of responsibility to meet all the needs of the community. Taylor began to experience anxieties and frustration from having a lack of knowledge as to what roles she needed to focus on.

Integrating the many roles the art therapist serves in community work (Ottemiller & Awais, 2016) is immensely difficult for a student who is at the beginning stages of professional identity development (Gibson et al., 2010; Skovholt & Ronnestad, 1992). The student can succeed in identifying and managing the roles, but combined with learning ethics and administrative tasks, much oversight and support is needed. The student may not disclose their struggles and end up feeling unsupported. Eventually back on campus we discussed ways to regain confidence by narrowing the scope of where in the community as a setting the student would flutter in with her approach.

History Center

In this third example of a community-based art therapy internship I assumed a voluntary role as an offsite supervisor for a student from another university than mine who forged a path into a prominent museum in Pittsburgh, PA. The intern, Jasmine, was familiar with my becoming an art therapist researcher (Moss, 2017) and our supervisory arrangement emerged years after I provided some consultation around securing art therapy internships in the city and program development. Assuming this site supervisor role was a shift in my usual role as academic supervisor. I got to experience supervision as an offsite supervisor in a community setting. My stake in the arrangement was two-fold: I was invested in Jasmine's development because she was creative and innovative, and I was afforded the opportunity to help pollinate an influential setting with art therapy.

We were delighted that the leaders in the museum who helped to foster the internship, the director of artifacts and the director of education outreach, were supportive, welcoming, and excited about innovative services. It was as if the perfect ingredients were present for a successful recipe, including Jasmine's academic supervisor having been formerly a museum-based art therapist. We shared language from our respective disciplines to help us acculturate and communicate ideas. For example, Jasmine was urged to substitute the word "exhibit" with "display" when proposing an art therapy interactive installation to museum departments because the former connoted issues of approval and funding and so on. Jasmine had nearly full reign over the massive facility and its affiliates to determine where and how she would apply art therapy. This was both inspiring and challenging.

The museum setting required Jasmine to take the position that community art therapy is both a setting and an approach, but we did not have the language to help guide us in our weekly supervision. I suggested that Jasmine identify her purpose and intention as a community art therapist, much like identifying her theory of change as a therapist. I again deferred to family systems language for joining and assessment. As Jasmine joined this community system, we identified micro, meso, and macro definitions of the museum community as a participant or client. Jasmine observed different floors and exhibits on different days of operation to get a sense of rhythm and flow of visitors. City sports and culture events impacted attendance and energy levels. Jasmine set up engagement activities in various spots in conjunction with exhibits to examine and relate with how patrons interacted and responded at points.

In our supervision Jasmine expressed confusion and anxiety about working in such a large space with seemingly unclear boundaries. I normalized her challenges with boundaries and anxieties of that of new art therapists (Moon, 2003; Moss, 2017; Moss et al., 2014; Skovholt & Rønnestad, 2003). The family, like a community, is an organism made up of parts and relationships and interactions. Drawing from my art therapy and family systems training and supported by literature about the use of metaphor in supervision (Awais & Blousey, 2020; Fish, 2008; Sommer et al., 2010), I spontaneously called the institution a "whale" to help Jasmine manage the system and its roles inherent in her work. Containing all the parts in a whale allowed Jasmine to assess the strengths, needs, resources, and readiness of the organization (Ottemiller & Awais, 2016). The whale metaphor as containment permitted Jasmine to freely move around inside the whale, learning about how it operated, how the parts were dependent, independent, and affected one another without the pressure of feeling as if she had to understand its enormity. Reducing the exponential movement of dynamics from the floors, exhibits, staff, docents, patrons from the city to beyond oceans, histories, individual interactions, departments, agendas, and artistic responses to one mammal created manageability and something to join with. Jasmine began to see parts of the community distinctly, even if fleetingly, and gave herself permission to focus and play.

Successful activities in this internship included community drawings on white boards, activity tables, completing sentences, making one's mark, and take-a-pause-and-reflect stations. Jasmine provided interactive stations while she was on site and for display when she was not on site as if to maintain art therapy presence.

As Jasmine learned to navigate the social realm that felt liberatory to her, she experienced interactions with patrons that activated countertransference related to social issues. This setting was a history center filled with exhibits about immigration, war, labor, slavery, Indigenous displacement, and contemporary cultural icons. Jasmine invited art therapy experiences with all who entered, including senior elders, international patrons, local families, and so on. One charged experience was particularly impactful when an elder white man, who was a United States veteran of the Vietnam War, initiated discussion about an exhibit of a military vehicle, one that he used to operate when he was on active duty. The interaction brought up concerns of racialized generational war trauma for Jasmine who is an Asian-presenting young woman, as well as topics of scope of "treatment" in the social space. Along with managing issues of countertransference in supervision, we explored Jasmine's ideas for art therapy opportunities that invited meaningful expressive co-creation in response to social issues.

Guided by supervision, Jasmine developed a process that was inspired by participatory research methods and included her personal art media of baking and making portrait cookies as a form of social justice. She recognized the experience and wisdom of the dedicated docents who had served the museum for decades. She set up interviews and made cookie portraits of them. In her interviews she listened to their experiences of serving the museum, losing their leader, and adjusting to new museum staff, and they shared their legacies. Her interviews and cookie portraits culminated as storytelling and display in conjunction with the museum holiday festivities. Docents and staff reported that they learned about each other and shared meaningful moments when reading their stories.

I believe that my experience with program development, art therapy education, and supervision and internship coordination made me uniquely positioned to provide supervision. The internship was only four months long, so there was not much time to establish rapport among stakeholders. We had shared vision, and all parties, including Jasmine, had seasoned professional experience. I knew how to advocate for Jasmine's needs with the museum. Though I could not know the outcome, due to my professional experience I could piece together knowledge and envision structure amidst the ambiguity and seemingly unclear boundaries in a setting where community art therapy was not yet defined.

Conclusion

Often art therapy internships lead to positions for art therapists once they have graduated. Interns are finding paths, managing systems, and showing communities what art therapy can look like. In campus supervision, interns in community sites reported feeling more confused when they listened to their peers' experiences of applying theory to practice in clinical settings. Perhaps a clearer definition of community art therapy would provide a framework. Leadership opportunities and employment are outcomes of the preceding examples. Each of these examples were circumstantial and unique and required networking, communication, and professional risk-taking. Challenges remaining are issues of adequate funding and post-graduate supervision.

References

Awais, Y. J., & Blousey, D. (2020). *Foundations of art therapy supervision: Creating common ground for supevisees and supervisors.* Routledge.

Deaver, S. P. (2012). Art-based learning strategies in art therapy graduate education. *Art Therapy: Journal of the American Art Therapy Association, 29*(4), 158–165. https://doi.org/10.1080/07421656.2012.730029

Fish, B. J. (2008). Formative evaluation research of art-based supervision in art therapy training. *Art Therapy*, *25*(2), 70–77. https://doi.org/10.1080/07421656.2008.10129410

Gibson, D. M., Dollarhide, C. T., & Moss, J. M. (2010). Professional identity a grounded theory of transformational tasks of new counselors. *Counselor Education and Supervision*, *50*(1), 21–38.

Lewis, J. A., Lewis, M. D., Daniels, J. A., & D'Andrea, M. J. (2010). *Community counseling: A multicultural-social justice perspective* (4th ed.). Cengage Learning.

Moon, B. L. (2003). *Essentials of art therapy education and practice*. Charles C Thomas LTD.

Moss, D. C. (2017). *The art therapist's professional developmental crisis: The journey from graduation to credentialing*. Mount Mary University.

Moss, J. M., Gibson, D. M., & Dollarhide, C. T. (2014). Professional identity development: A grounded theory of transformational tasks of counselors. *Journal of Counseling and Development*, *92*(1), 3–12. https://doi.org/10.1002/j.1556-6676.2014.00124.x

Ottemiller, D. D., & Awais, Y. J. (2016). A model for art therapists in community-based practice. *Art Therapy*, *33*(3), 144–150. https://doi.org/10.1080/07421656.2016.1199245

Skovholt, T. M., & Ronnestad, M. H. (1992). Themes in therapist and counselor development. *Journal of Counseling and Development*, *70*(4), 505–515. https://doi.org/10.1002/j.1556-6676.1992.tb01646.x

Skovholt, T. M., & Rønnestad, M. H. (2003). Struggles of the novice counselor and therapist. *Journal of Career Development*, *30*(1), 45–58. https://doi.org/10.1177/089484530303000103

Sommer, C. A., Ward, J. E., & Scofield, T. (2010). Metaphoric stories in supervision of internship: A qualitative study. *Journal of Counseling and Development*, *88*(4), 500–507.

Chapter 4

Centering Relationship

Education and Supervision Considerations for Working in Community

Emily Goldstein Nolan, Erica Brown, and Yasmin Tucker

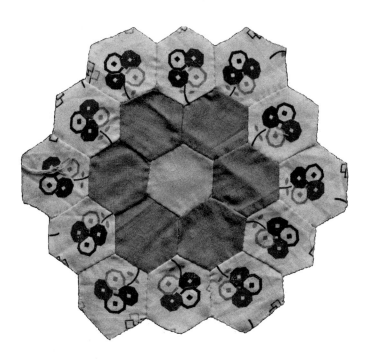

Honeycomb quilt block 4

Introduction

Art therapists, art therapy educators, and art therapy students have been work-ing in communities since the beginnings of the field. Many art therapists started in school communities, such as Edith Kramer and Lucille Venture and others, while Irene Champernowne, Cliff Joseph, Sara McGee, Georgette Seabrooke Powell, and Rita Simon, were working in greater community contexts through

DOI: 10.4324/9781003193289-4

community healing and social empowerment (Black Smith, 2014; Doby-Copeland, 2019; Gipson, 2019; Hogan, 2001; Joseph, 2006; Kramer, 1951; Stepney, 2019; Venture, 1977). I (Emily) have learned so much from these visionaries and think of them as ancestors who continue to guide the evolution and types of art therapy community work.

As an art therapist I have engaged with communities using art therapy over the last 20 years while also teaching and supervising graduate art therapy students. Most recently, I have had experiences in restorative circles that have informed the way that I teach and engage in supervision with art therapists and art therapy interns. In the restorative practice experiences, I began to see how important it is to first build community and trust with one another and let the work flow from there. I view working with students from a community perspective, in that we build relationships with one another in the classroom in a way that is supportive, empowering, and challenges each other. In weekly group staff meetings at Bloom Art and Integrated Therapies, Inc. in Milwaukee, we attend to one another in the group first, meaning that we meet as people first. Each person checks in with how they are doing, what is impacting them, what they are excited about, what they want to share, and they can ask for what they need from the group. Then the members of the group attend to each other's needs. Sometimes the needs are to discuss clients, or to explore a situation that is happening in one of the many community art therapy services on and off site. Sometimes the needs are to be supported while integrating difficult insights or sharing ways that we each engage in self-care.

This chapter focuses on supervision and education in community, ways to examine and reflect on the self in relation to the community, which effectuates ethical practice and widening the view of what is included in community practice.

Art Therapy Supervision

In my experience as an internship coordinator for two different graduate art therapy programs in the United States I have seen that an effective field placement provides opportunities for students to engage in supervised experiences of art therapy while also challenging their existing mental models of art therapy practice, beliefs about themselves, and the people participating in art therapy services. Overall, "reliable and accountable supervision supports not only the art therapist, but also directly influences the experiences of the people engaged in art therapy" (Awais & Blausey, 2021, p. 8.) Field placements in the community is one context where ideas, skills, and knowledge come together for art therapy students, and they see how what they have learned impacts the participants.

In the United States students are required to amass a number of field place-ment hours under the supervision of a site supervisor and a faculty supervisor. Once an art therapy student has graduated from a program, they are respon-sible for accumulating additional practice hours beyond their master's degree to become registered and board certified. The hours beyond their degree also require supervision by an appropriately experienced and credentialed mental health professional and/or art therapist. In several states there is additional abil-ity to become licensed as an art therapy or related professional; each state has varied requirements. Credentialing requirements around the world differ and some areas have no credentialing or educational requirements. Regardless of location and licensing, it is a good critically reflexive practice for any art thera-pist to be in regular contact with others who are engaged in community work, a supervisor, or to consult with peers.

Awais and Blausey (2021) provide a thorough general guide for art therapy supervision. Further, several types of supervision are outlined in the art therapy literature, such as the mentor model and integrative developmental model (Moon & Nolan, 2019; Thomas, 2010); art-based models (Fish, 2017; Miller, 2012) and models for art therapists working within specific populations such as those seeking help for addictions (Chilton et al., 2020), in hospices, (Potash et al., 2015) and via long distance communication (Orr, 2010). In training and as new art therapists, supervision is an imperative part of the developmental process. Even seasoned therapists benefit from supervision or consultation as they enter unfolding relationships that unearth challenges at any time. Within supervision, art therapists dedicate time and space to reflect on their thoughts and actions within sessions, and thereby deepen their understanding of their clients' needs and how to appropriately respond. Within the supervision session the supervi-sor provides an outside perspective that invites the therapist to understand how their own experiences and contexts influence their reactions and interactions with their clients.

Various people are involved in art therapy supervision, whether it is tied to a field placement, or the art therapist is working to complete their hours for cre-dentialing. The people include the student or the new art therapist, the faculty supervisor when working in a school program, the site supervisor who primarily is at the setting or focused on the work of the setting, and the participants. Each individual plays an important role in the training of the art therapist.

Awais and Blausey (2021) wrote, "a genuinely effective supervisor creates a reassuring and supportive environment for the art therapist's field experience" (p. 8). The interaction works best when the supervisee can explore responses and reactions in a shame-free environment (Thomas, 2010.) I have learned that the experiences that supervisees don't want to talk about are the ones that they should be talking about the most. The best supervisors are aware of their own identi-ties, and practice with cultural awareness, fluency, and humility. The supervisor understands the community perspective, is educated about the community the supervisee works in, or has had experiences with that community. The supervisor models how to create multiple successful relationships and is aware of how they relate to others. The supervisor creates space for supervisee learning, meeting, and interacting with them regularly.

Community Art Therapy Supervision

When addressing community art therapy and supervision, a varied mix of knowledge, skills, and traits are important to treat as benchmarks. *Before* working in the community, the art therapist should demonstrate the following baseline characteristics and skills: (Stoltenberg & McNeil, 2009)

- **Interpersonal skills:** the ability to listen and be empathic with others; respect for/interest in others' cultures, experiences, values, points of view, goals and desires, fears, etc. These skills include verbal as well as nonverbal domains. An interpersonal skill of special relevance is the ability to be open to feedback;
- **Cognitive skills:** problem-solving ability, critical thinking, organized reasoning, intellectual curiosity, and flexibility;
- **Affective skills:** affect tolerance; tolerance/understanding of interpersonal conflict; tolerance of ambiguity and uncertainty;
- **Self-regulation skills:** to understand one's own bodily reactions to stress, and to be able to ground oneself while still connected to self and others;
- **Personality/attitudes:** the desire to help others; openness to new ideas; honesty/integrity/valuing of ethical behavior; personal courage;
- **Expressive skills:** the ability to communicate one's ideas, feelings, and information in verbal, nonverbal, artistic, and written forms;
- **Reflective skills:** the ability to examine and consider one's own motives, attitudes, behaviors, and one's effect on others;
- **Personal skills:** personal organization, personal hygiene, appropriate dress.

I have found that *before* working in the community supervisees should have knowledge about:

- Assessment and interviewing;
- Appropriate art therapy tasks and directives with knowledge of art supplies and media;
- Group facilitation knowledge and experience;
- Ethical and legal concerns;
- Individual and cultural differences (ICD):
    - Knowledge and understanding of what it means to work with people across cultures and experiences;

- Understanding of one's own situation, (e.g., one's ethnic/racial, socio-economic, gender, sexual orientation; one's attitudes towards diverse others) relative to the dimensions of ICD (e.g., class, race, physical disability etc.);
- Understanding of the need to consider ICD issues in all aspects of art therapy work (e.g., assessment, treatment, research, relationships with colleagues, etc.);
- Self and other awareness (cognitive and affective), one's motivation (intrinsic *vs.* extrinsic validation, willingness/ability to navigate complexity), and autonomy.

Even with the described skills in place prior to engaging in art therapy in the community, I have seen that art therapists need space and time to maintain critical reflection. In most programs, graduate student interns are required to meet with their supervisors regularly, having ample time to discuss and explore topics. At Bloom, we meet once a week for an hour in staff meetings, the interns meet for an additional hour with their supervisor, and outside of those sessions the interns use a visual journal to explore their concerns and interactions visually and aesthetically with clients and the community.

Some examples help show how supervision with the lens of community art therapy skills and traits can work. I once worked with a graduate art therapy student who was an art therapy intern at a shelter for unhoused people. She was a white, educated, cisgender female in her mid-20s, and was planning to introduce a new project to the community in the next studio session. She used supervision to discuss her idea for the directive. She wanted to have each person create a house using a similar house structure that she created. We discussed her reasoning and thought process behind working with the topic of home and providing a structure for each participant. Moreover, using questions, not judgments, we deconstructed her values to determine that she thought that everyone should have a home, and if they were able to dream about it, they could make it happen by manifesting it. In supervision we explored what we knew about the participants at the shelter and named what we didn't know. We did not know that everyone at the shelter wanted to have a home, or that they agreed that a home takes on the structure she was looking to provide. We unpacked the idea that because someone had a dream, they had the ability to make the dream happen. She concluded that her efforts could potentially place her own values of what home is onto the community and serve to dislocate her as an ally. We explored other ways for her to explore more general topics that could encourage people to find their own sense of shelter, safety, and security. She used her visual journal to discover more about her own personal values and how they related to the community she was working in.

In another example, an intern came to supervision and reported that she had been late to her internship that day because she had locked her keys in the car with the milk inside. Trying to get the car open made her late to the community art therapy studio at the shelter. She described that she was frazzled as she unlocked the doors to the studio and there were lots of people waiting for her outside the door. She let them into the studio and was complaining about her situation. One man said, "Well at least you have a car and the money to buy milk!" She agreed with him and immediately knew this was something she needed to explore further in supervision, but first used her visual journal to process the experience. In addition to thinking about her identities (similarly, a white educated cisgender female in her mid-20s), and the power she held in her position as an intern, we worked through identifying boundaries and personal disclosure, and understanding and exploring how she presents to others in each space.

Art therapy supervision in the community is tripart, including the art therapist, the art therapy supervisor, and the community. I have been at my best as a supervisor when I am open to working with students in a non-shaming way that offers support and feedback. When students and practitioners have been authentic, open to incorporating feedback, and aware of self and others, they report feeling the most integrity from doing the work. The following offers an example of how art therapy is conducted in a community art therapy internship at Bloom Art and Integrated Therapies, Inc in Milwaukee, Wisconsin.

A Model for Community Art Therapy Supervision

Working from a liberatory and attachment framework while sustaining critically reflexive art therapy practice (Kapitan, 2010), I conceptualized a way for art therapy interns who work in community services to understand interpersonal relations and support healthy relationships in the community art therapy studio. The intention is to use intrapersonal knowledge and interpersonal clinical skills to identify how the participants operate in the world and relate to others. People engage with one another in different ways based on their previous experiences in relationships, and this knowledge supports how I see the studio as a place of belonging. I encourage the interns to interact with and support the participant interactions in a meaningful way that encourages inclusion. It is important to note, however, that art therapy exists and is implemented in myriad ways, which include a wide array of community practices. Supervision in community art therapy can be applied differently depending on the needs and context of the community.

Relationships and the Community Art Therapy Studio

When working in community art therapy studios with an understanding of interpersonal connection, the studio can play a role in fostering healthy relationships and functioning.

While the client and I talk and make art, which are explicit processes, we are also engaging in the implicit processes of neurobiological communication. "Regulation theory thus describes how implicit systems of the therapist interact with implicit systems of the patient" (Schore & Schore, 2008, p. 14). From a self-regulated place, I offer my clients an opportunity to engage in a safe, secure, reliable relationship. If dysregulated, we can co-regulate by bringing our nervous systems and emotions into balance. The therapeutic relationship can positively influence future intrapersonal, interpersonal, and community relationships.

People's trust in others can be jeopardized by experiences of trauma, especially experiences of relational trauma; therefore, engaging in community can help a client heal. As an art therapist, I attend to relational needs within community-based models by providing opportunities to experience safety, structure, and outlets for expression and relating. Pat Allen (personal communication, December 22, 2020) conceptualizes that in the community art therapy studio, the art therapist's artist self moves to the foreground and the therapist self moves to the background. People come together in art therapy sessions where the participants engage in healthy relationships, and people can feel a sense of belonging in that community (see Figure 4.1).

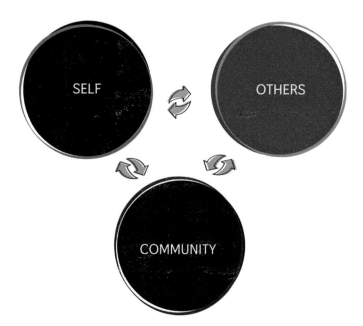

Figure 4.1 Multidirectional influence of the community art therapy experience

The community studio is a microcosm of the larger community that ideally provides support for a just, loving, diverse, and stimulating, creative experience for all its members. Healthy relationships are the foundation of art therapy experiences, which resonate on the individual and the community level.

In this approach, as an art therapist I seek to occupy a non-oppressive standpoint that does not support pathology-based hierarchies. I have developed an understanding, through supervision and a critically reflexive art therapy practice (Kapitan, 2010), that a pathology-based diagnosis is not necessary to provide therapy intentionally and effectively. The insight is that all studio participants are living out their attachment narratives in their interactions with others in the art studio. As an art therapist, I can bring my artist self forward, to ground myself and then pay careful attention to the behaviors and dynamics of the relationships within the studio. As I perceive the dynamics, I am intentional in my own actions and interactions to promote healthy relationships and nervous system regulation.

The Supervision Framework

All the participants in the community art therapy studio, including the art therapists, have a history of relationships with themselves, others, and their artwork and artmaking process. In this framework, the art therapists carefully attend to the structure of the studio, choosing materials, art tasks, and experiences to offer, often with collaboration from the community. As keepers of the space, the art therapists are reliable and on time to open the space. They are continually aware of their own nervous system regulation and how they show up to do the work. Within the studio, the art therapist and the participants collectively create studio rules that all agree to follow, and the art therapist encourages participants to encourage, accept, and support each other. The art therapy studio is consistent, regularly addressing the needs of the community.

As a supervisor, I encourage that art therapists and art therapy interns understand the following concepts:

1. **Art therapists engage in critical reflection to center their practice in community minded concepts.** Community work has its own approach that considers the whole. One intention of supervision is to provide avenues to explore the art therapist's own identity as a form of self in relation to their community, maintain humility, and understand participants and communities in their whole context. Art therapists are supported while examining their own actions and interactions with community members in the studio and consider their own role as a community member.
2. **Community members welcome each other into the space each day.** Another intention of supervision is to consider that welcoming each other to the studio supports the creation and maintenance of a positive community.

This initial experience is repeated each time the studio opens to create a sense of reliability and trust within the community as a ritual and orients one another toward shared purpose and values. As a parallel process, art therapists are welcomed into supervision and engage in a similar orientation to that of the weekly session.

3. **Community members provide a safe and reliable studio environment for one another.** Another intention of supervision is to support the art therapist as they understand how a safe and reliable studio environment functions. The art therapist makes sure that the studio is open as scheduled when access is easiest for the community. The community of artists create the rules for working in the studio and respecting the shared space. The implicit communication between the members of the studio intentionally promotes nervous system regulation and healthy connections with self, others, and the art.

4. **The studio is filled with materials for exploration, experimentation, regulation, and play.**
   Another intention of supervision is to support the fact that the art materials available encourage artistic inquiry, with ample time for the community to discover new ways of creating, play, and, if desired, use materials for self-regulation. The art therapist shares their artistic skills, practice, and knowledge with the community freely. The art therapist may share art instruction or other knowledge with the community, and the community members are invited to share their skills and knowledge as well.

The following examples illustrate how this supervision framework has been used in supervision in the community art therapy studio. In the first vignette Erica outlines using the framework to supervise art therapy graduate interns and reflects on how she has experienced and observed this model of supervision in student development. In the second vignette, Yasmin Tucker, a former intern, shares her experience of training within this model.

COMMUNITY ART THERAPY SUPERVISION FRAMEWORK REFLECTIONS

Supervisor Reflection: Erica Browne

I (Erica) have experienced this supervision model in multiple settings and roles. My first encounter was as an art therapy graduate student during my first internship. Post-graduation, I sought out the same supervision style with Emily as I acquired hours toward licensure. I now supervise interns through this relational model.

As an art therapy intern, I was equally as eager to practice art therapy in the studio with participants as I was to learn more about myself as a novice practitioner. In supervision, I was encouraged to explore the relationship with my artist identity. I began to view the art I created as relational objects with insights that can guide and support treatment with individuals and groups. This is how my art and art therapy practice developed a dynamic relationship with one another. All elements of art therapy became relational to me. My supervisor, Emily, helped guide this self-reflection and discovery that fueled my own theory-based graduate research and my art therapy practice today that includes both individual and community-based work.

As a supervisor this reflexive approach informs everything I do. Establishing a relationship of confidence and trust is at the core of this supervision model. For predictability, I am sure to be consistent with time, location, and expectations. We begin with a brief orientation to ground into the space and five minutes of artmaking using any materials with the prompt of: "What are you bringing to supervision today?" This open-ended question allows the intern to bring in recent successes in the studio, areas of curiosity and growth, where they might be struggling with a client, or personal life issues that may be impacting their ability to provide art therapy at the time. Interns are encouraged to reflect on these experiences to facilitate awareness about themselves as new art therapy professionals. This process also allows them to experiment and be vulnerable around other interns and the supervisor, further establishing trust and safety. Usually, we will end the supervision by adding or changing the artwork created earlier in the session. This practice allows the intern to integrate any insights, form acceptance around an issue, visualize the change or resource needed, and identify their strengths.

When encountering the inevitable insecurities and curiosities that come with learning to be an art therapist, I present the intern (or myself sometimes) with the statement I heard again and again as a supervisee: "Make art about it." This encourages creative self-exploration and validates the essential relationship with the artist identity to work through challenging narratives that our clients present with. I've learned that the continued investment in my art practice makes me a better artist, supervisor, and art therapist. This helps me maintain regulation and facilitate an emotionally safe and supportive environment for studio participants or my clients. There is no separating the relational approach that informs my practice.

Intern Reflection: Yasmin Tucker

As a second-year graduate art therapy student at Mount Mary University in Milwaukee, WI, I (Yasmin) completed my first clinical internship at a drop-in center for unhoused people during the spring of 2015. I recall entering the room with my co-intern anxious to perform at my best and remember every word of what I learned in school so far. I quickly realized that the organic nature of the drop-in studio asked more of my authentic self than my polished academic self. As clients entered the studio space, it was my role to create the ritual of welcoming, invite self-reflection, encourage creativity, and foster new relationships with each other—including the two bright-eyed interns.

I knew then that we (the interns) represented past teachers, spiritual leaders, treatment providers, sisters, cousins, aunts, mothers, missed opportunities of youth, and power dynamics to those we served. The open-ended nature of the community art studio allowed complete strangers to navigate their relationship with the world around them through art-play and -making. This model also facilitated an opportunity for all of us to try, fail, and try again in a nourishing environment that we created completely unscripted.

One of the most memorable moments during this clinical placement was with an adult client/artist in his late 20s with low intellectual functioning, a history of traumatic brain injury, chronic homeless, and social neglect. He indicated that his mother welcomed him back into their family home due to his participation in "school." What he called "school" was the twice-a-week art therapy group held at the drop-in center. Our weekly open studio provided him with meaningful activity and a place to demonstrate his phenomenal painting and mix-media arts skills. The open studio invited him to rewrite the narrative about his intellect, talents, and overall potential. I recall thinking, "Wow, he is amazing and what an honor it is to shine in the same space at the same time."

During weekly supervision, I would express my frustration in navigating my in-between roles: one where I served Black and Brown people who looked and lived like me, juxtaposed with the mostly white ivory tower of higher education that I took the city bus to, four hours a day, four to five days a week. I felt, at the time, a compulsory loyalty to the client/artists within central-city Milwaukee, and an internal pressure to reject my academic community, which I knew I belonged to and I loved.

As I processed the dual roles with my supervisor, I observed my range of creativity and flexible thinking broaden. I began to embrace the "yes, and" motto of being a part of both worlds, rather than having to choose one or the other. With this, I began to develop confidence in my ability to circumvent the persistent yet narrow thought that I do not fit in (with family, with peers, with myself). As I developed trust in my supervisor, I was able to express my truth and irritation with poverty, racial inequality, lack of representation in higher education, and the extreme segregation in Milwaukee. I became less intimidated by the stories of resilience and regret I heard at the drop-in center.

The safety in our supervision relationship allowed me to model it to the client/artists during my internship. Long term, this semester represented some of my first experiences of accepting all parts of me. The zesty, mildly insecure, gregarious, thick madame, urban, clapback, leader, innovator parts, and everything in between.

The Self and Identities in Relation

Identity is not static but dynamic, dimensional, and fluid. Identity contains experiences of gender, age, race, ethnicity, social class, status of wealth, physical ability, sexuality, education level, geographic location, religion, language, etc. Figure 4.2 conceptualizes identity through intersectionality. Intersectionality is the dimensions of identity that interconnect and cross over one another and how overlapping social identities relate to systems of oppression, domination, and marginalization (Crenshaw, 1989; Talwar, 2010).

Individual and Community Member

In general, individuals make up communities. In one way, when I (Emily) work with an individual who then goes out into the community and engages with others, this influences the greater community. Conversely, when I work in

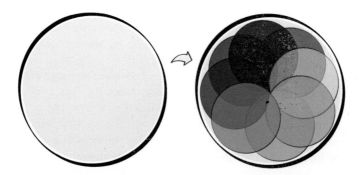

Figure 4.2 Differentiating identity made up of intersectional components. Each color circle within the larger circle represents one component of a person's identity

communities, I am also working with individuals, but my outlook regarding the person and the approach to the community changes. Together we decide what goals to work toward and then take actions to effect transformation. Although the target of change is the community, and not the individual, the individual will grow too.

Within the community art therapy studio, participants can explore an artist's identity. Forming a relationship to art and exploring that relationship within the context of the therapeutic community in the studio facilitates the formation of an artist identity (Moon, 2002). The artist identity can be contrary to labels such as *homeless*, *drug addict*, *mentally ill*, and so on, that participants may have personally experienced and are reinforced outside of the art therapy studio through societal stereotyping. Along with the formation of an artist's identity, Allen (2008) wrote that "the healing aspects of artmaking arise from the making and doing, the trying and failing, the experimenting and succeeding, alongside others" (p. 11). Making art and relating to the artwork and others within a community studio can help a participant develop freedom from a fixed idea of self, providing an opportunity for personal and collective transformation and healing, while being in the presence of others who are committed to similar exploration.

One central element I have witnessed in the community art therapy studio is freedom. The participants make an active choice to engage in art therapy through the community studio. They are not designated/assigned to an art therapy group based on their admittance to a hospital or because of a particular diagnosis. Rather, the studio is offered to the public or a specific group of people, and participants choose to take part. In addition, participants are free to choose what materials they would like to work with and what projects they might like to work on.

Because it is outside the dominant narrative of treatment, not a hospital or outpatient program, the community art therapy studio can also be an access point for engaging in art therapy that is more appealing or accessible to participants. The community art therapy studio Bloom invites participation on one's own terms, and therefore further encourages empowerment. The therapeutic work within the community art therapy studio is not part of a treatment plan, and it is not directed by anyone other than the participants with the support of an art therapist. I see that this makes an opportunity available to explore therapy in a less intimidating or overwhelming environment.

Art Therapy Practitioner and Community Member

As an ethical practitioner who works in community, I constantly consider my own assumptions of people, power, institutions, and communities. Ethical practice and challenges in the community will be covered in more depth in Chapter 5. As an art therapist, I develop both intrapersonal and interpersonal skills for working with clients. However, working in community contexts shifts my view and use of my skills from the individual to a global level. This perspective shift from the micro view to the macro view was difficult for me at first, but I realized it is not unlike how I look for patterns, both effective and ineffective, in client and family functioning. Additionally, the skills of working with individuals and groups are the basic building blocks of working with communities. With the turn from individual to group to community, dynamics become more complex.

As a master's level student in art therapy, my focus was learning how to be in relationship with someone and how that could help them create the change that they wanted in their life. The program I attended was not overly focused on diagnosis. As an Adlerian student, I learned to diagnose, but, in some ways, I felt that I was a detective discovering the client's patterns of being in the world, holding space for them while they tried on new behaviors, and helping them to regulate their nervous system to deal with difficult feelings and emotions. I was very focused on individuals and families for the first ten years of my art therapy career. As I gained experience, I realized that I was missing important components of influence in the lives of my clients. I began to search for information that could widen my view of the client experience and what they were bringing into their sessions with me.

I went through the Freirean process of conscientization, (Friere, 2012) where I began to critique and reconstruct my own practice (Prilleltensky & Nelson, 2002), gaining awareness of what happens for clients in the contexts of the larger system and the institutions present within it. I began to challenge my own assumptions about my work with clients, how I was trained, and how I taught and supervised students. What happened was that the power dynamics that seemed invisible to me before my intentional critical reflection began became visible. I saw that clients were facing more than I thought when they entered my therapy office. Specifically, how their experiences within systems and affiliations to cultural and social groups influenced what my clients were experiencing emotionally (see Figure 4.3).

Both therapists and clients have power within therapeutic relationships and in everyday life. However, therapists always have power over their clients, even in community contexts where power is thought to be more shared. Prilleltensky and Nelson (2002) outline "three primary uses of power, 1) power to strive for well-being, 2) the power to oppress and 3) the power to resist marginalization and strive for liberation" (p. 7). Both individuals and communities can be powerful. A person's and a community's potential for power considers both ability and the opportunity within social and historical circumstances to enact agency. Considering power is necessary in understanding social identity, culture, and developing cultural fluency (Abrams & Moio, 2009).

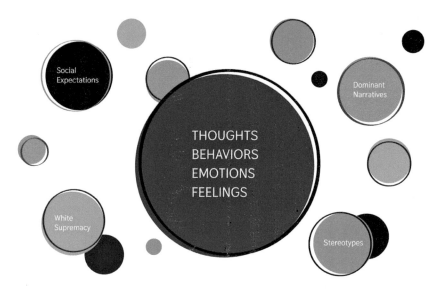

Figure 4.3 Internal and external influence. This provides a visual depiction of internal oppression, thoughts, behaviors, and feelings, and external oppression, such as social expectations, dominant narratives, and stereotypes

Cultural Humility

Having awareness of my own identity has grounded me in working with those whose identities are both similar and different to mine, which keeps me focused on practicing with cultural humility.

Jackson (2020) wrote,

> cultural humility is a derived set of principles that offer grounding for cultural awareness. It is a skill set and a state of being that can offer a way to engage in critical cultural discourse. It is not a one size fits all and may be difficult for some to absorb and cultivate. It is a way of developing a worldview with integrity and respect for oneself and those one works with. It can bring dignity to those who have felt stripped of their sense of self as well as lending empowerment to those whose voices have been denied witnessing. It offers a tangible way to enter into dialogue when tensions are surmounting all sense of reason and hope.
>
> (p. 7)

According to Inoue (2007), several ideas are key to committing to cultural fluency. As an art therapist, I strive to continually attend to each of these ideas coupled with critical self-reflection as a responsible community member.

- Tolerance of ambiguity (my ability to accept lack of clarity and to be able to deal with ambiguous situations constructively);
- Behavior flexibility (the ability to adapt own behavior to different requirements/situations);
- Knowledge discovery (the ability to acquire new knowledge in real-time communication);
- Communicative awareness (the ability to use communicative conventions of people from other cultural backgrounds and to modify my own forms of expression correspondingly);
- Respect for differences (curiosity and openness, as well as a readiness to suspend disbelief about other cultures and belief about my own culture);
- Empathy (my ability to understand intuitively what other people think and how they feel in given situations).

An addition to developing the ideas presented above is the skill of learning to decenter whiteness and mainstream tendencies. Decentering is a metacognitive process and is included as a critical part of reflexive practice (Bernstein et al., 2015; Hitchcock & Flint, 2015). I see that most policies and institutions in America have been developed from a predominantly white male perspective. When I have located myself in relation to my clients and community it helps me as the art therapist to then locate the mainstream and white perspective and examine how it is operating. That insight into the larger dominant paradigm sheds light for me on the lived experiences of those who don't live inside that narrative. To be an ethical, effective, culturally responsive clinician, I try to be aware of power dynamics and the stigmatizing experiences of those from historically marginalized groups (Ancis, 2004). This requires first creating an awareness of my own experiences and then recognizing that this experience is only one against many possibilities. Decentering urges my curiosity and engagement, keeping the relationship central and relying on hope and belief that stronger communities are possible only in partnership with the voices and needs of the people in the community.

Understanding cultural humility, fluency, and intersectionality requires my lifelong process of self-reflection, self-critique, and self-reflexivity (Talwar, 2010). I realize that I do not arrive at cultural humility; there is no endpoint as identities and social locations can change over time with new experiences. Rather, cultural humility takes my active engagement, addressing power imbalances, and seeing individuals and communities as experts in culture. As I practice community art therapy with humble awareness, I recognize the dynamic nature of communities and culture and how culture can be influenced over time depending on location. Initially, "since the therapist … is the agent of change in individual-led interventions, training must start with the individual" (Prilleltensky & Nelson, 2002, p. 69). As an art therapist who understands my own identities, I can view those I work with

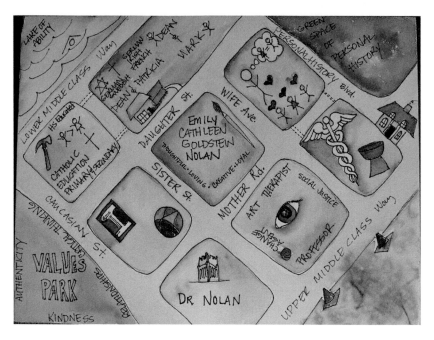

Mind map of my intersectional identities. I created this while reflecting on my own intersectionality in 2017. Creating this map visually helped me to understand my own history and the current ways that I hold power in my life. I use this knowledge of myself to understand and mindfully interact with others, intentionally engaging in meaningful ways

as complex, intersectional humans with multiple experiences of external and internal struggle with the right to strive for well-being.

Conclusion

Supervision has been an important component in the development of art therapists and can be specialized to work in community art therapy practice. As an art therapist, I have worked to develop intrapersonal and interpersonal skills, and then widened my perspective to include a relational aesthetic view of community. Central to my work in community is knowing my own identity, upholding the community as an expert, understanding cultural differences, and practicing cultural humility while developing cultural fluency. I seek to understand contexts and how the community interacts with systems and institutions in society and how people hold and wield power.

Art Experience

Circle Context: Art Experience for a Group or Learning Community

1. Individually, draw a circle on a piece of paper. Outside the circle draw a representation of who you are on the outside: for example, your culture, family, history, values. Inside the circle draw something that represents who you are on the inside: your thoughts, feelings, and behaviors. Cut the circle out.
2. Get with a partner and discuss your circles. Do not consider anything outside the circle; only the thoughts, behaviors, and emotions represented inside the circle.
3. With your partner, discuss the whole picture, with the circle and surrounding area.
4. Reflect:
   • How much and what were you able to learn about your partner from just the circle?
   • How much and what were you able to learn about your partner from the whole picture?
   • What have you learned about the importance of considering the person and their whole context?
5. Discuss what you experienced and learned about context with the learning community.

References

Abrams, L. S., & Moio, J. A. (2009). Critical race theory and the cultural competence dilemma in social work education. *Journal of Social Work Education, 45*(2), 245–261.

Allen, P. (2008). Commentary on community-based art studios: Underlying principles. *Art Therapy, 25*(1), 11–12. https://doi.org/10.1080/07421656.2008.10129350

Ancis, J. (Ed.). (2004). *Culturally responsive interventions: Innovative approaches to working with diverse populations.* Brunner-Routledge.

Awais, Y., & Blausey, D. (2021). *Foundations of art therapy supervision.* Routledge.

Bernstein, A., Hadashm, Y., Lichtash, Y., Tanay, G., Shepherd, K., & Fresco, D. (2015). Decentering and related constructs; A critical review and metacognitive processes model. *Perspectives on Psychological Science: A Journal of the Association for Psychological Science, 10*(5), 599–617. https://doi.org/10.1177/1745691615594577

Black Smith, M. (2014, June 9). At the feet of a Master: What Georgette Seabrooke Powell taught me about art, activism, and the creative sisterhood. Truthout. https://truthout.org/articles/at-the-feet-of-a-master-what-georgette-seabrooke-powell-taught-me-about-art-activism-and-the-creative-sisterhood/

Chilton, G., Lynskey, K., Ohnstad, E., & Manders, E. (2020). A case of El Duende: Art based supervision in addiction treatment. *Art Therapy*. https://doi.org/10.1080/07421656.2020.1771138

Crenshaw, K. (1989.). Demarginalizing the intersection of race and sex: A Black feminist critique of antidiscrimination doctrine, feminist theory and antiracist politics. *University of Chicago Legal Forum*, *140*, 139–167. https://chicagounbound.uchicago.edu/cgi/viewcontent.cgi?article=1052&context=uclf

Doby-Copeland, C. (2019). Intersections of traditional healing and art therapy: Legacy of Sarah E. McGee. *Art Therapy*, *36*(3), 157–161. https://doi.org/10.1080/07421656.2019.1649548

Fish, B. (2017). *Art-based supervision: Cultivating therapeutic insight through imagery.* Routledge.

Freire, P. (2012). *Pedagogy of the oppressed.* Continuum.

Gipson, L. (2019). Black Women's consciousness in art therapy. In S. Talwar (Ed.), *Art therapy for social justice: Radical intersections* (pp. 96–120). Routledge.

Hitchcock, J., & Flint, C. (2015). *Decentering whiteness.* Center for the Study of White American Culture, Inc. https://www.euroamerican.org/public/decenteringwhiteness.pdf

Hogan, S. (2001). *Healing arts: The history of art therapy.* Jessica Kingsley.

Inoue, Y. (2007). Cultural fluency as a guide to effective intercultural communication: The case of Japan and the U.S. *Journal of Intercultural Communication*, *15*, 1–13. https://immi.se/intercultural/nr15/inoue.htm

Jackson, L. (2020). *Cultural humility in art therapy: Applications for practice, research, social justice, self-care, and pedagogy.* Jessica Kingsley.

Joseph, C. (2006). Creative alliance: The healing power of art therapy. *Art Therapy*, *23*(1), 30–33. https://doi.org/10.1080/07421656.2006.10129531

Kapitan, L. (2010). *Introduction to art therapy research.* Routledge.

Kramer, E. (1951). *Art therapy in a children's community.* Charles C Thomas.

Miller, A. (2012). Inspired by *El Duende*: One-canvas process painting in art therapy supervision. *Art Therapy: Journal of the American Art Therapy Association*, *29*(4), 166–173. https://doi.org/10.1080/07421656.2013.730024

Moon, B., & Nolan, E. (2019). *Ethical issues in art therapy* (4th ed.). Charles C. Thomas.

Moon, C. (2002). *Studio art therapy: Cultivating the artist identity in the art therapist.* Jessica Kingsley.

Orr, P. (2010). Distance supervision: Research, findings and considerations for art therapy. *The Arts in Psychotherapy*, *37*(2), 106–111. https://doi.org/10.1016/j.aip.2010.02.002

Potash, J., Chan, F., Ho, A., Wang, X., & Cheng, C. (2015). A model for art therapy based supervision for end-of-life care workers in Hong Kong. *Death Studies*, *39*(1), 44–51. https://doi.org/10.1080/07481187.2013.859187

Prilleltensky, I., & Nelson, G. (2002). *Doing psychology critically: Making a difference in diverse settings.* Palgrave Macmillan.

Schore, J., & Schore, A. (2008). Modern attachment theory: The central role of affect regulation in development and treatment. *Clinical Social Work Journal*, *36*(1), 9–20. https://doi.org/10.1007/s10615-007-0111-7

Stepney, S. (2019). Visionary architects of color in art therapy: Georgette Powell, Cliff Joseph, Lucille Venture, and Charles Anderson. *Art Therapy*, *36*(3), 115–121. https://doi.org/10.1080/07421656.2019.1649545

Stoltenberg, C., & McNeil, B. (2009). *IDM supervision: An integrative developmental model for supervising counselors and therapists* (3rd ed.). Routledge.

Talwar, S. (2010). An intersectional framework for race, class, gender, and sexuality in art therapy. *Art Therapy*, *27*(1), 11–17.

Thomas, J. (2010). *The ethics of supervision and consultation: Practical guidance for mental health professionals.* American Psychological Association.

Venture, L. (1977). *The Black beat in art therapy experiences.* Unpublished dissertation, Union Institute (formerly Union Graduate School).

Chapter 5

Ethical Practice and Challenges in Community

Emily Goldstein Nolan and Kai Ying Huang

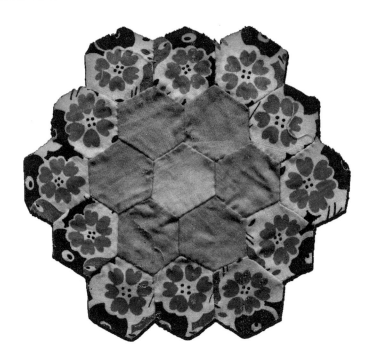

Honeycomb quilt block 5

Introduction

In Chapter 4, I discussed important concepts to consider when training to work in community art therapy practice settings; I see that ethical practice and training are intertwined in that chapter. As Park (2019) noted, "understanding the cultural context within which an individual lives is, therefore, crucial for any teaching or therapy to be effective; not to do so would not just be uninformed

DOI: 10.4324/9781003193289-5

practice, it would be unethical practice" (p. 70). Here, Chapter 5 describes how art therapists can commit to ethical practice and face challenges when working in community and navigating complexity. This is not meant to be a comprehensive manual for ethical practice in community art therapy—that would be beyond the scope of this book and would require considering many different legal practices and cultural norms.

Overall, ethical practice is not black and white. My graduate students always seem to want concrete answers to what is ethical or not in individual practice, and my only consistent answer has always been that it is not OK to have a romantic or sexual relationship with any clients. In communities, ethical practice is no different. Communities are complicated and require art therapists to be critical of their actions while carefully navigating unfolding relationships, shared decision-making, and goals. Ethical practice requires that art therapists understand the rights communities have and that following best ethical practices is their responsibility to both the community and to society (Corey et al., 2019).

Art therapists are required to abide by the standards set forth in the areas in which they are practicing or that may be developing as art therapy develops in that location. My perspective in writing this book and chapter is as a cisgender, white, middle class, female art therapist who lives and practices in Milwaukee, Wisconsin, in the United States. Before writing this book, I co-wrote an ethics book with Bruce Moon, (Moon & Nolan, 2020); however, that book focuses on the legal issues and ethical practice of art therapy in the United States. A section of that book very briefly discusses ethics in the community art therapy studio and does so from a US perspective. This chapter is informed by the literature, the experiences of those who work all over the world, and my own perspectives. However, I am certain there are ethical issues, concerns, and challenges that art therapists experience in community that I do not cover within this chapter.

Who is the Client?

Art therapists who work in and with communities face many challenges. One challenge can be logistic: How to engage participants, where to hold the artmaking sessions, what materials are available, and knowing the artistic skill level the participants hold. One additional challenge that arises when working in community is determining who is included when defining the client.

In community art therapy, the client is the community. Who is included in the community and the types of community can be controversial, and what Cathy Moon (Personal communication, June 30, 2021) called "slippery." This topic of what and who makes up a community is covered more in depth in Chapters 1 and 2, as community is a setting *and* an approach in art therapy practice. But one of the largest challenges is that community can include the participants, the art therapist, and the funders, and resources (see Figure 5.1). In speaking with many art therapists across the globe during the interview process for grounded theory,

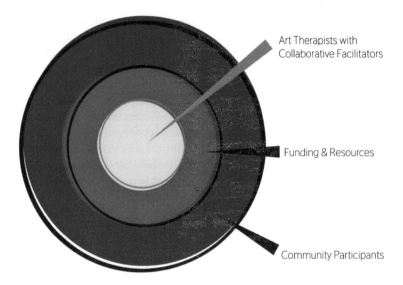

Art Therapists with
Collaborative Facilitators

Funding & Resources

Community Participants

Figure 5.1 The client

it became clear that even if the funders did not participate in artmaking or other activities that they funded, they were a stakeholder in that community with goals that needed to be attended to, for, and with, the community participants.

Timm-Bottos (1995) described that before starting the community art studio, ArtStreet, located in Albuquerque, New Mexico, she collaborated with local leaders, including a local medical provider who worked with unhoused people. That collaboration with the studio invited potential funders into the space and ArtStreet subsequently received continued funding, keeping the nonprofit mission alive. ArtStreet was funded through collaborative efforts among community members and leaders. However, when the funder is not a local community member or the funding source isn't directly physically, socially, or financially integrated with the location of the community art therapy program, project, or workshop, this can be challenging for a community to reconcile.

Funding

In the United States, organizations that engage in community work can be public, private, nonprofit, or for-profit (Corey et al., 2019). For-profit institutions usually provide a fee-for-service; nonprofits can do this as well, but also apply for grant funding. When initially creating Bloom in Milwaukee, Wisconsin, I considered whether I should create it as a nonprofit or a for-profit. I met with a local university's free legal clinic for nonprofits to consult about Bloom's organizational structure. I investigated the costs for organizing Bloom as both a nonprofit and a for-profit. However, I realized the startup costs for creating a nonprofit were significantly higher. I also made the connection that many grant funders reside in the 1% of the population that hold the most wealth; I questioned how their interests could align with folks who needed and wanted community services. I decided to open Bloom as a for-profit business because at the time I could not fathom how I could continuously search and apply for grant opportunities. At first being a for-profit business structure gave Bloom the most flexibility; a lot of the work at Bloom was fee-for-service with private clients and some contracts with community agencies for art therapy. I questioned this decision as being too idealistic, but for the first ten years of existence, as a certified woman-owned business Bloom had been able to work with nonprofit organizations and get funding without nonprofit status. After ten years, as the community art therapy initiatives grew, Bloom converted to a nonprofit. The organization is now eligible to apply for grant funding while offering needed services to the community and jobs to art therapists. Bloom gains funding for community projects through private donors, grants, and contracts with organizations for art therapy services.

Every founder's assessment and decision will be different. Effective practices indicate that art therapists and collaborators in community endeavors work with funders who have goals that align with the community, and partners should provide evidence in support of the attainment of those goals. No one within a community is more important than another; however, each member has a goal, role, and place; and that needs transparency, recognition, and fulfillment.

Art therapists have described that finding funding often presents a challenge. Many nonprofit art therapy agencies are small, and the art therapists are doing much of the work to facilitate art therapy sessions, network, and develop programming with the community as well as find funding. I find it can be especially challenging not having roles for people within the art therapy organization that support fundraising alone, and yet everyone in the organization as well as outside supporters need to work together to support sustainability.

Program Sustainability and/or Sustainability of Support

Long-term sustainability involves drawing from the social, environmental, and economical resources readily available to start and maintain community art therapy endeavors. Before opening a community art therapy studio at the shelter for unhoused people, I thought a lot about sustainability of services, but I lacked some understanding of long-term sustainability. Initially, I wanted to make sure that the studio experience was offered consistently for the members of the shelter, a few times per week, to address mental health concerns. The shelter also provides health and wellness services to the members through an attached free clinic. Members would sign up for a spot to see a volunteer nurse or physician when they needed. My thought process was that if needed, the free clinic would be available for services if the therapists were not on site when needed. The studio at the shelter was open for ten years and was facilitated by art therapy graduate students. However, thinking about long-term sustainability of that studio, the shelter was not able to partner in providing resources for supervising graduate interns, or the administrative costs of facilitating the studio, nor did Bloom have support at that time for finding funding. Without a plan for the continuation of the program and the costs to run it, although running for ten years, the program closed.

As another example, art therapist Ana García led online art hives for Spanish speakers throughout the coronavirus pandemic. She understood the limited resources and from the start promised the community she would lead the art hive for a year. She was intentional with the online community in communicating the expectations for program duration. She reported that once the program ended, she focused on her own self-care, securing additional funding for future art hives, and supporting others who host online art hives. In her view, even when programs end, there is space for new ideas and options.

Reyes (2019) discussed the importance of sustainability of support over the novelty of providing help through art therapy when working in communities after a natural disaster. She questioned the local resources available to support the community beyond any initial community art therapy intervention. In her experience there is a natural tendency to "over support" initially when a disaster impacts a community, but the retreat of that support leaves the community without services to continue healing, causing further harm.

I see that to avoid leaving a gap that potentially harms the community once services are withdrawn, art therapists and community collaborators can ask:

- What services are available outside of the art therapy/community program that is offered? If so, how can art therapy support the connection of the community to those services?
- How are services funded?
- What other environmental or social resources are available?
- What will the community need long-term?
- Will support from this endeavor create dependence or interdependence?

Culture and Scope of Practice

"Culture—with its beliefs, customs, and loyalties—is inseparable from ethical practice because one's perspectives and decisions are based upon the way one lives in the world, as shaped by the society to which one belongs" (Park, 2019, p. 76). Ethical practices that are culturally relevant understand the collectivist or individualist facets of the communities in which the art therapist works. "Art therapy is a discipline which develops according to the particular social, cultural and economic circumstances of individual countries" (Gilroy, 2000 in Stoll, 2005, p. 6, p. 190). The engagement in ethical work requires that one understands many components of the culture and community being practiced in, which can include:

- Knowing the limits of the location of art therapy training as within or outside of the community and location of practice (Berman, 2019; ter Maat, 2019);
- Whether art therapy is a field with recognized credentialing in that area;
- If it is appropriate within the community's context to train citizen leaders to conduct art therapy (Berman, 2019);
- Identifying the cultural art practices that are already embedded within the community that can be brought in to address the concern (Alfonso, 2019);
- Knowing why the art therapists are present (Vivian, 2019);
- Knowing whether the art therapist is an insider or outsider within the target community (Vivian, 2019);
- Questioning if art therapy and psychology is developing alongside a longstanding tradition within the culture to honor spiritual healing interventions (Vivian, 2019);
- How to navigate complexity and role flexibility in therapeutic situations (Corey et al., 2019).

These considerations and questions seek to guide art therapists in applying critical thinking to community practice. At its best, community art therapy supports, empowers, and celebrates communities.

Ethical Considerations for Defining Scope of Practice

Many benefits of practicing in community exist. When working collaboratively in and with communities, the scope of art therapy is highly nuanced and many ethical standards of art therapy practice and helping professions the world over contain some premise that the therapist use ethical decision-making as a member of the community. If newly practicing, it is expected that the therapist or helping professional seek supervision with a practitioner that has experience in that setting. My thoughts are that in the case of community art therapy this expectation is similar; however, art therapy is not a universally recognized profession worldwide, and people don't always have access to graduate-level training programs in their location. Each geographical location of practice has its own set of ethical standards, or an emerging set of standards based on the culture's values and systems present and the practice of those who are conducting art therapy services. A dynamic interplay exists between the evolution of ethical standards and the active practice of community art therapy by those therapists doing the work. Taking responsibility for the evolution of practice and what is included is itself an ethical act.

Impact of Training and Licensing

To restate an important point, art therapy is practiced all over the world but is not yet a recognized field in each location. Often, when a field is not recognized as a formal profession, such as psychology or psychotherapy, and is developing, there is not a training program in that location. Art therapist Donald (2019) wrote that she relied on her credentials from the United States to prove legitimacy for the discipline of art therapy while working in the West Indies. Many art therapists seek training outside of their geographical area and then bring art therapy back to integrate their learning into the culture and health system. Depending on where the therapist trains and the values (implicit or explicit) of that training, the therapist is in a bit of a conundrum. For example, art therapists are often trained with US and UK ideas of applying theory to art therapy practice. With globalization, it is difficult to say that cultures and countries wouldn't already be influenced by Western ideals; however, the art therapist must know the lens that they see people and their work through and that will be influenced by the values of the training they attended.

Additionally, art therapists who are sole practitioners, or one of a few in their location where there is not a recognized field, can often become the person to guide and supervise others well before they have gained needed experience. Donald (2019) wrote,

> The first ethical issue I encountered arose from the assumption that my education and credentials granted me insurmountable knowledge about all topics related to mental health. As the only mental health professional at my workplace and the only art therapist in the nation, I unwittingly became the go-to person for complex cases for which I was mostly unprepared.
>
> (p. 112)

Julia Volonts, who practices art therapy in Latvia, noted that as a new professional with master's-level US training, she is often tapped for ethical consultation by other mental health professionals and is helping to set a standard of ethical practice in her locale. She consistently encourages herself, and those who consult with her, to be self-reflexive and ask, "Am I causing harm?" (Personal communication, April 19, 2021). The relationship between ethical practice, conscious self-inquiry, and humility with the intent to do no harm seems to be key as practice evolves worldwide.

The following is a reflection on practice written by Kaiying Huang that highlights her experience as an art therapist trained outside of her practice location.

BEING A SOJOURNER ART THERAPIST WORKING IN COMMUNITY IN TAIWAN

Kaiying Huang

As a Taiwanese-born art therapy sojourner, someone who studied in the United States and then returned to practice and teach in my homeland, I (Kaiying) hope this reflection can facilitate exchanges of cross-cultural awareness surrounding issues in ethical practice in different parts of the world.

Transplantation of the Western Discipline

Compared to the way in which art therapy is established in the United States and the United Kingdom, art therapy in many Asian countries is a recent profession. Taiwan is one of the earliest places in East Asia to have introduced art therapy and established professional organizations (Wolf Bordonaro, 2016). Over the past two decades, art therapy has gained popularity via Western guest speakers and Taiwanese sojourners who bring their Western training home. Although the first graduate-level art therapy program was established at University of Taipei in 2005, it has continued to be the single art therapy master's degree education provider in Taiwan. The enrollment statistics (see Figure 5.2) indicate that more people are submitting enrollment applications for the entrance examination, while the number of students accepted into the art therapy program remains the same. Overall, due to the lack of well-established art therapy higher education training, individuals still seek their art therapy training overseas.

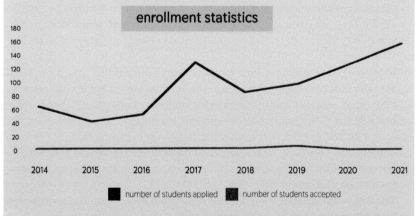

Figure 5.2 Enrollment statistics for an increasing number of students applying to the art therapy program in Taiwan

After sojourner art therapists complete their training abroad and return to home countries, many understand their local and indigenous worldviews, but there may be a dissonance between those worldviews and their Western art therapy training (Carliér & Salom, 2012; Park, 2017; Solomon, 2006). On the other hand, in Taiwan, the faculty in the art therapy program are all trained in the United States, where the training is highly influenced by psychodynamic thinking. In the Chinese domain of art therapy literature, cross-cultural understanding of culturally specific approaches to contemporary Chinese communities are relatively new and limited. The direct transplanting of Western art therapy knowledge that has occurred in Taiwan may impede the indigenization process that would have allowed its culturally appropriate adaptation to serve a rapidly changing Chinese society.

Hence, rather than completely relying on understanding the clients' mentalities from a Western paradigm of individual psychological development, Taiwanese art therapists highlight the importance of considering the ethical applications of art therapy from cultural perspectives (Huang, 2021). Specifically, approximately 96% of Taiwan's population is ethnic Chinese. Under the influence of global Westernization, modernity has had a great impact on people in Taiwan; however, respecting the superior is still a fundamental principle in social interaction among Taiwanese people (Yang, 1995). Within the therapeutic context, Taiwanese art therapists have encountered hierarchical dynamics within the early therapeutic alliance, and their clients tend to respect the therapist as an authority figure and have an intolerance of structural ambiguity (Huang, 2021).

Similarly, when interacting with others, traditional Chinese values promote a modesty orientation, which advocates using an implicit communication style for the purpose of maintaining interpersonal harmony. Chinese people can typically refrain from displaying strong emotions publicly (Hwang, 2009). Thus, in group settings, fear of losing face, a high level of self-consciousness, and impulse control are the common clinical challenges faced by Taiwanese art therapists when engaging people with non-directive and spontaneous artmaking (Huang, 2021). In practice, art therapists should be aware that the traditional teachings of Confucius may reinforce Chinese clients' tendency to think that learning self-expression is a waste of time (Chong & Liu, 2002).

In consideration of clients' inner structure influenced by Confucianism, Chinese people view themselves as interdependent with their social groups (Markus & Kitayama, 1991); art therapists must shift to a client-in-context perspective to examine the therapeutic rationales and consider whether art therapy interventions are congruent with clients' social realities. After years of working with clients who are relatively strongly affected by Confucian relationalism in Taiwan, I have learned to apply an educational approach by teaching artistic skills and utilizing playful art activities. The playful activities help to loosen their formalistic social behaviors, which can increase confidence in artmaking and decrease collective shameful feelings that arise from sharing personal experiences within their collectivist social context.

Moreover, the pervasive social stigma associated with mental issues among Chinese populations has been documented in the literature (Hwang et al., 2006). As mentioned earlier, the Chinese cultural traditions place great importance on family; therefore, a person who talks about family issues may risk disrupting social harmony (Hodges & Oei, 2007). The therapist may sometimes provide a more pragmatic psycho-educational intervention in a solution-focused and didactic approach to strengthen the therapeutic relationship and reduce shameful feelings during the early stage of therapy.

Challenges to Ongoing Sociopolitical Changes

Another practical factor in the unique help-seeking attitudes with Taiwanese clients is health insurance coverage. In 1995, a low co-pay system with mandatory enrollment was instituted by the government. Although psychotherapy and counseling has developed rapidly along with economic acceleration, non-psychiatric counseling is still not covered by the government's insurance. Under the Taiwan's National Health Insurance Act, only psychiatric counseling performed by psychiatrists and clinical psychologists in hospital settings can be covered by the National Health Insurance (NHI). Even when public psychotherapy treatment is covered, people often wait months to receive a short consultation due to limited resources. In respect of insurance coverage, the public mental health resources are mainly directed toward traditional medical treatment due to limited resources, while out-of-pocket cost for other forms of psychotherapy in a private clinic is relatively expensive. Consequently, clients who seek psychotherapy services in those facilities where the costs are not covered by the NHI tend to expect goal-oriented, cost-effective, and time-limited approaches in treatment.

Fortunately, in recent years, the Social Affairs Bureau in Taiwan has recognized the importance of psychotherapy as a viable solution to psychological problems. For example, in the field of domestic violence, a client who is within the government social administration system can receive free short-term counseling via referral from their social worker (Shen, 2001). With the support of government subsidies and partial private funds, there are a few domestic violence nonprofits and charities that provide long-term counseling with the co-pay fees that are set on a sliding scale based on a client's income.

My cross-cultural clinical practices enable me to see not only that different health care systems could influence the theories and approaches utilized by therapists, but also that the pre-existing systems could impact the scope of art therapy service. In order to be eligible to practice psychotherapy in Taiwan, individuals need to hold valid national psychology licensure as established by Taiwanese Legislature rather than certification or registration by professional organizations. Under this condition, in recent years, some Taiwanese creative art therapists have actively been participating in the licensure policy-making process. However, before art therapy was introduced to Taiwan, over the last 20 years a gradual reform of education and legislation in the field of counseling and clinical psychology had been happening. Creative art therapists have faced challenges in the process of establishing a national licensing system by trying to fit into the existing governmental licensure system. Like the experiences of art therapists in a number of countries, without achieving independent art therapy legislation by the government in Taiwan, this would leave limited opportunities for art therapists, especially, when working in public education and the governmental social welfare system. Consequently, people seeking psychological help often exclude art therapists as mental health professionals. Taiwanese art therapists often face the challenge of how the public understands their professional role and experience unstable employment in the years following graduation or returning from study abroad (Chang, 2021). Since there are very few full-time jobs with the title of art therapist in Taiwan, a certain number of art therapists work in many different settings to achieve a stable income. Establishing community art therapy service, I found it is necessary to elevate the professional status of the art therapist while I cultivate trusted relationships with my colleagues and funders in different settings. My practice working with families experiencing domestic violence has taught me that no professional can deal with the complexity of trauma alone. The work of community art therapy can effectively address the practical problems with the lack of access to mental health service covered by NHI. Via referral by a social worker, domestic violence clients who are in need of psychotherapy can participate in art therapy groups as an integral component of the community-based welfare service. In order to provide a more effective and sustainable quality of service, in practice, I have learned to embrace a more proactive communication by collaborating with related professions as well as networking and strengthening relationships with administration in the health care system.

As mentioned above, under the influence of Confucian relationalism, one's willingness to share resources and the expectation of obtaining aid from others corresponds to the closeness of the relationship one has with them (Hwang, 2012). According to my experiences, sometimes, many organizations I worked with prefer a favorable relationship with a therapist over professional abilities and credentials. In consideration of Chinese thoughts for favoring the intimate and reciprocity, it takes time to cultivate mutual trust relationships and build partnerships with multiple professionals from the different backgrounds. After years of working in Chinese communities, I have realized that developing a sense of belonging to professional networks and communities is a fundamental step in providing high-quality, culturally effective art therapy practice.

Summary

In sum, when art therapy discipline is transplanted from the West into a new country, both art therapy practice and the establishment of art therapy in that country are influenced by cultural, political, and economic forces. Regarding ethical practice within changing cultures, art therapists should not overlook the importance of achieving comprehensive cultural insight and should be aware of the ongoing sociopolitical conditions. Practicing appropriately in the context of the culture in which one is working is imperative to the ethical practice of art therapy.

Training Non-Art Therapists

As art therapy develops and evolves globally, access to master's-level training programs isn't always possible. To meet the needs of a location that does not have art therapy or training, art therapists can determine if and how it is ethically appropriate to train non-art therapists to provide art therapy services through task shifting and sharing (Keshri & Garg, 2021; Orkin et al., 2021). Community art therapists collaborate with many different types of practitioners: social workers, psychologists, psychiatrists, artists, performers, and so forth. Art therapists must carefully consider how knowledge of art therapy processes are shared with community practitioners. And as art therapy develops communities of practice and practitioners outside of US and UK notions and standards, those communities of practitioners can be trained in culturally appropriate ways that are sensitive to the nature and goals of art therapy. Several art therapists have discussed the topic of training non-art therapists. In fact, the American Art Therapy Association (2013, 2016) offers the following best practices for training non-art therapists in American contexts:

> When providing training and/or supervision to non-art therapists, art therapists take precautions to ensure that trainees understand the nature, objectives, expectations, limitations and resulting qualifications of the supervision and/or training as distinct from formal studies in art therapy.

I would add that art therapists who are trained in the United States and work in other cultures should consider the lens through which they view art therapy and community as they train non-art therapists. Without considerable support, non-art therapists working in community art therapy processes may inadvertently dive into material that leaves community members feeling inappropriately vulnerable without being able to stabilize them, and may not understand art materials and their power, how to structure the studio and session, and how to curtail inappropriate interpretation of work. However, in areas where the field of art therapy is not recognized or licensed, using US standards may also not be appropriate (Kalmanowitz &Potash, 2010; Osei, 2019). Although art therapists are careful to not undermine the profession, or potentially cause harm to participants, training non-art therapists to conduct therapeutic art sessions can fill a need (McNiff, 1997; Moon, 1997). Additionally, Kalmanowitz and Potash (2010) note that offering art therapy training to other professionals can increase their skill sets and create recognition and awareness for art therapy.

I see that as art therapy emerges in areas all over the world, the ethics specific to those locations appear as well. Art therapists uphold and impart ethical practice in communities and training of non-art therapists, which includes relevantly adapting art therapy while upholding high practice standards. The standards incorporate teaching trainees to approach artmaking and communities sensitively and together the art therapists and the community establishes an appropriate scope of practice boundaries.

Paola Luzzatto (personal communication, July 6, 2021) created a training program in Dar es Salaam, Tanzania, through Muhimbili University. The program started in 2016 and prepares medical professionals in art therapy to work in the Open Studio model. At the time Luzzatto implemented the training program, there was very little, if any, art therapy in Tanzania. Luzzatto reported that she deliberately chose health professionals to maintain ethical practice because they would be more prepared in the event of a client or community member becoming destabilized. She worked with the trainees to "help them to become more aware of the areas in which they are not trained" (Kalmanowitz & Potash, 2010 p. 23), which in this case is art therapy. She decided a training program was best to educate health professionals and introduce art therapy as an additional skill. The training provided includes 50 hours of theory and practice and 50 hours of internship over an eight-week period. At the end of their training, the participants get a certificate as an "Open Studio Expert"; they do not call themselves art therapists. Luzzato is adamant that professionals maintain a non-interpretive framework of art therapy and practice under the supervision of an experienced art therapist.

Art therapists training non-art therapists globally consider all aspects of the system in that environment, including the educational and health systems, the culture, structure of professions, and practice. Art therapists training non-art therapists consider their experiences, providing supervision and ongoing support, educating about materials, exploring the complexities of interpretation, working with the image, and structure of sessions. Art therapists in any setting are always upholding the use of critical thinking in the application of art therapy in teaching, training, and practice (Kalmanowicz & Potash, 2010; Moon & Nolan, 2020).

Ethics of Boundaries and Navigating Multiple Roles

During my doctoral research examining community art therapy practice, as a part of action research and at the request of the participants at the daytime shelter for the unhoused, an intern accompanied two women on the city bus from the shelter to the art museum. On that bus ride, one of the women revealed that she had been raped the night before in an overnight shelter. She did not ask the therapist for help; she wanted only to have someone hear her story, to which both the therapist and other woman listened. Afterward, the intern called me to seek supervision regarding the young woman's disclosure and debrief the trip to the museum. We reasoned through both boundaries and the multiple roles of the art therapy intern within that experience.

Often in community art therapy the art therapist plays multiple roles and carefully navigates boundaries. Important to note is the distinction between a boundary crossing and a boundary violation. According to Corey et al. (2019) a boundary crossing is a departure from commonly accepted practices that could have a benefit for the participant, whereas a boundary violation is a rupture that results in harm and is unethical.

Because of the multiple roles people play in community art therapy, boundaries can be quite tricky. "Establishing clear professional boundaries requires both professional and personal sophistication and maturity, coupled with commitment to constant evaluation of art therapists' motivations and behaviors" (Moon & Nolan, 2020, p. 147). I have experienced this myself when working and supervising students in community, and many of the therapists I interviewed about their work in community also reflected that challenge. Art therapists hold a variety of responsibilities in community platforms (Moon & Shuman, 2013). The many roles that art therapists play in community contexts, such as facilitator, participant, funding seeker, manager, artist, supervisor, etc., make it challenging to address boundaries but it is always up to the therapist to make sure that those roles do not cause harm to participants. Therefore, it is the responsibility of the therapist to be self-reflexive and know if they are proceeding unethically. Rozanne Myburgh, who works at a community creative arts therapy organization Lefika La Phodiso in Johannesburg, South Africa as the managing director and a drama therapist, noted that she is transparent about the roles she plays to address role flexibility (Personal communication, July 12, 2021). Role flexibility is the balance of all the roles that the therapist plays across the services offered (Corey et al., 2019.) Myburgh discussed that she manages the multiple positions she holds with the community as she transitions to a new program or area. In whatever role she is functioning at that time she states, "this is who I am now …, this is where I am now ..., and this is what we are doing now ... ." This helps her to clarify the boundaries for not only the participants, but also herself.

My youngest child, Jasper, is an artist and a maker. Since he was very little, he has craved getting his hands into art materials, loves to figure out how things work, and explores the limits of what he can do creatively. When I first started the community art therapy studio at Bloom, he would beg me to take him each Saturday. The graduate interns facilitated the studio, so in that space and time I would be a participant among the other artists. I carefully reasoned through my decision to attend the studio session with Jasper. I considered what might happen if some of my individual clients attended the studio and saw me making art alongside them with my son. I clarified that I was there as a participant, I did not attend to the needs of the participants in the studio. I shared as appropriate and was reflective of my presence in the space. A few of my individual clients did attend the community studio as participants, and later in our individual sessions they revealed even more about their concerns as parents. "When handled appropriately, multiple relationships do not need to disrupt the therapeutic encounter. In fact, when managed well, they can even strengthen it." (Potash, 2019, p. 196). Seemingly, my clients' view of my interactions with my child deepened their appreciation for me as their therapist and as someone who understands what they might be experiencing with their own children. I think that art therapists who work in community can develop role flexibility, tolerating ambiguity while maintaining critical self-reflection that mitigates causing harm to participants.

When people with different backgrounds, views, and experiences are present in community, people can experience conflict depending on how those ideas are expressed. In my experience, working in community requires effort in managing my awareness of myself-in-relation to others, and acknowledging both my values and biases. Others can say and do things that I wouldn't say or do or that strike a particular nerve with me given my own past experiences and sense of self. I remain mindful and ask myself:

- Who am I and what role am I playing in this space?
- What does their behavior tell me about myself?
- What is this person bringing out of me that I need to work on for myself?
- What might this person be seeking that the community can provide?
- Is how I am responding to this person something that promotes their sense of belonging?

Record-Keeping

In individual, family, and group art therapy sessions, practitioners are required to keep clinical records. In community art therapy experiences this may happen depending on how the sessions have been presented and what has been communicated about art therapy to the participants. The art therapist determines:

- What records need to be kept;
- How consent to treatment is obtained;
- How participants understand confidentiality and the limits.

At the heart of this question is the challenge of determining how art therapy is included in the program execution and communicating that to the community. This is traversed with intention and transparency but can be complicated because art by its nature allows the flexibility of providing therapeutic services in a non-stigmatizing way. But disguising *treatment* through artmaking is deceptive. Therefore, negotiating power is essential and relies on the therapist sharing power with the community. The art therapist critically reflects on how the community understands art therapy and what the art therapist's role is in the program, project, or work.

A standard of what records are kept in the practice of community art therapy is not fixed. Art therapists place focus on what records are kept and how, and which are established as relevant to the context and culture of the community and the art therapy program within it. Moon and Shuman (2013) wrote about their experience with ArtWorks in Chicago, IL, where initially the parent organization that housed the program required written progress notes for each participant served at the agency. However, Moon and Shuman pushed back, arguing that writing notes would differentiate those participants from other ArtWorks participants who did not receive services at the parent organization. What resulted was that the organization conceded, and no case records were kept for ArtWorks. Overall, art therapists apply critical thinking when determining the records and the processes of record-keeping and communication. The question is: What type and depth of record-keeping serves the goals of the community-as-client and the individual simultaneously, but where the priority is decidedly not "individual treatment" but rather a therapeutic community art therapy experience that ripples out in multiple ways?

Consent to Treatment with Children

At Lefika La Phodiso, Berman (2019) wrote that she often experienced children wandering into the studio to make art without a parent present to provide consent. Although the studio welcomed the children, Rozanne Myburgh (Personal communication, July 12, 2021) also noted that at Lefika they have developed a process of sending a consent form home with the child. The parent can send a text photo of the signed consent back to a WhatsApp number. The child can attend three sessions before they must have the consent signed by a parent to attend. At Bloom, under Wisconsin law, anyone 14 years of age or older can sign consent for medical treatment themselves. As a result, at the all-ages community art therapy studio, Bloom allows children 14 and older to attend without parent presence or consent, and with a parent when the child is 13 and younger. Every legal jurisdiction may have varying regulations or laws that impact choices about obtaining consent for child participants in community art therapy.

Safety

Establishing physical and emotional safety with participants is a foundation of ethical practice in any helping profession. In art therapy, therapists intentionally consider the place of practice or where programming will occur. In community contexts, the art therapist ensures that the environment is conducive to artmaking, that there is adequate ventilation for the materials being used, that they have knowledge of material hazards and potential toxicity, that there is access to water, and that the location is private to ensure the confidentiality of the group (Moon & Nolan, 2020.)

Outside of the logistics of the setting where art therapy happens in community, a thorough assessment of the resources the community has available for follow-up care is necessary and happens simultaneously and continuously. Several of the art therapists I interviewed discussed developing programming targeted toward wellness especially if the community wouldn't have further opportunities beyond the program offered for long-term care. Leara Glinzak works in community with the Traveling Loom Project. She built a loom on wheels, bringing it to different areas of Grand Rapids, Michigan, aiming to bridge connections between neighborhoods. She was careful to have people sign a consent form to participate, but also thoughtfully structured the project so that people contributed to the community tapestry through words, colors, or images. She found that often people would stop to talk. She was careful when opening a space of sharing, contemplating peoples' experiences, the potential for the disclosure of trauma, and poking at a wound (Personal communication, June 29, 2021.) Similarly, Linhn Guyen works in Vietnam providing community art therapy in collaboration with local NGOs. She, too, cautiously develops programming and structures her sessions focusing on awareness, wellness, prevention, and resilience rather than exploring trauma or using depth psychology (Personal communication, June 24, 2021.) Both of these therapists were very aware of the long-range impacts the experience could have on participants and the limitations on the community's follow-up resources and they carried this ethical mindset from the beginning of the projects.

Art and Craft Materials

Art and craft materials are the tools of creative expression, ritual, healing, and transformation. Choices of materials are vast, from mainstream options such as paint and pencils to found objects and other non-traditional media people have most accessible. Practitioners in the community setting seek out materials that the community will feel successful using, paying attention to the age level and abilities of the members. General ethics would implore that art materials are chosen with input from the community, attention to accessibility, and an assessment of what is available. Practitioners observe what creative materials and processes are used in the community already that will be relevant to the participants' daily experiences and cultural practices (Alfonso, 2019). I see that the art and craft materials used in community art therapy sessions are available as resources in the community.

When I attended art therapy graduate school in the early 2000s, I was taught the importance of using quality professional materials that invited people to perceive artmaking as important. The accepted idea was that adults might feel demeaned by using childlike materials and if provided "real" artist supplies then adults would take art therapy seriously. Over time, I let go of the notion that the art materials used with participants had to be mainstream and moved toward a view that if any item was used creatively as an art material, anyone could be an artist. My socially constructed beliefs about the "right" art materials (Leone, 2021) were ruptured, and I saw that the idea of artist and artmaker became more accessible. My work in the shelter with unhoused folks provided evidence, as the artists there used all sorts of donated items to make art. I found that fixating on the art materials can get in the way of innovation, play, respect, acceptance, and empathy.

Exhibiting Artwork Ethically

Morris and Willis-Rauch (2014) wrote that participating in an art show and exhibiting work can attend to the goals of artistic empowerment, collaboration, and reducing stigma. In their experience, providing social action art therapy in a hospital using a community approach, exhibiting artwork was seen as a form of communication and a chance to share with the viewer and wider public about the experiences of the hospital community. Therefore, the wider community becomes witness, and art therapy participants are offered additional opportunities to be seen. When art is exhibited in the community, whether from a community art therapy initiative or as part of someone's experience in an individual art therapy session, the opportunity for communication with the community is present, and is another way for the participant(s) to feel a sense of belonging in that community.

However, when art is taken from the therapeutic context and made public through exhibition, the art can be subject to interpretation and meanings that the artist did not intend to be possible (Leenstra et al., 2014, p. 228.) The artwork can be misconstrued, and that can cause the participant to have both good and bad responses. Conversations and shared decision-making within the community are necessary to ensure that everyone understands the intent or purpose of the exhibit (Vick, 2011) and the risks (Moon & Nolan, 2020).

Garlock (2019) wrote the following questions to engage in critical decision-making when considering exhibiting artwork.

- Where does the work come from?
- Are there consent forms?
- Are they comprehensive and understood by the signer?
- What does the art look like?
- In what context was it created?
- What is the purpose of showing the work?
- How does showing the work affect who made it?
- Who benefits from showing it?
- What or whom does it promote?
- Is it for sale and, if so, who gets the money and how is it distributed? (p. 141.)

In my view, because of the complexity of public discourse on almost any subject, heightened by the nature of community art therapy and those who participate, the ethical planning and execution of exhibitions works best when it is as collaborative and participatory as possible.

Media

As art therapy is practiced in more visible and public settings, the media can easily become interested in sharing stories of art therapy with their audience. Television, radio, podcasts, news stories and the like are ways to widen the potential community of art therapy participants, providers, and funders. Media attention furthers awareness of art therapy and its many benefits; this can help to secure funding to both begin and sustain programs. Talking with folks who practice all over the world, often what comes into fashion through popular culture and media coverage can often be the focus of what projects get funding. However, art therapists bear the responsibility for how the message is conveyed and how the impact of that message intersects with the art therapy community. Art therapists and community members can collectively decide what is shared, but it is always the art therapist's responsibility to foresee any harm that may come to the participants resulting from media coverage and bring those concerns to the community.

Obtaining Advice

Part of professional ethics typically involves the ability to consult advice as well as to be self-reflexive. This occurs in addition to, or at a level beyond, the supervisory component of training. In areas where art therapists are licensed, they may have access to an ethics hotline or other resources where matters of concern can be discussed, often anonymously. The American Association of Art Therapists has an ethics committee, resources, and an inquiry process (2017). In areas without licensure or a strong regulatory body, art therapists may form cohorts of practice among themselves, sharing dilemmas or concerns in a space of trust and candor among a few individuals, or communities of practice. Sometimes, legal advice is the best course of action. In any case, seeking outside advice for community art therapy ethical practice is important.

Conclusion

This chapter has focused on the challenges that art therapists face when practicing ethically in community-based endeavors. Questions that arise include how community is defined, who is included in community, and concerns with funding and sustainability. As art therapy expands globally in practice areas, scope of practice and the training of non-art therapists for community art therapy becomes a central issue of concern. Art therapists employ critical thinking in all ethical decision-making. Ethical practice in the community art therapy context involves determining what records to keep, if any, how art therapy is framed to the community, the safe use of materials and keeping of confidentiality, consent for minors, exhibiting artwork, and engagement with media.

Art experience

Creating Role Flexibility: Individual Art Experience

Use any blank archetype image, visually explore all the roles that you play in community. Reproduce the image as needed to match the number of roles. Then maybe choose one or two other members of your community, and create images to match their roles. Cut them all out and arrange them visually, exploring the following:

How do these roles overlap and intersect?
How might they hinder the work of the community?
How might acknowledgment of them enrich community work?
Are there any roles I may be ready or willing to let go?
How is art making involved in navigating multiple roles?
What boundaries are in place to keep everyone safe?
What boundaries could be strengthened?
What influence do I have on my community members?
Overall, what did you learn from this experience?

Creating Role Flexibility: Community Art Experience

Use any blank archetype image provided here to visually explore all the roles that you play in community. Reproduce the image as needed to match the number of roles. Have each member of the community use the blank archetype to depict the roles they play in community. Arrange the figures visually for all to see. Discuss the roles together.

References

Alfonso, M. (2019). After the typhoon: We brought art materials, they wanted coffee. In A. DiMaria (Ed.), *Exploring ethical dilemmas in art therapy, 50 clinicians from 20 countries share their stories* (pp. 27–35). Routledge.

American Art Therapy Association. (2013). *Ethical principles for art therapists.* American Art Therapy Association.

American Art Therapy Association. (2016). Art therapists training non-art therapists. www.arttherapy.org/ upload/ ECTrainingNonATs.pdf

American Art Therapy Association. (2017). Ethics inquiries. https://arttherapy.org/ethics/

Ballbé ter Maat, M. (2019). Culturally adapted art therapy practice: Is it ethical? In A. DiMaria (Ed.), *Exploring ethical dilemmas in art therapy, 50 clinicians from 20 countries share their stories* (pp. 50–54). Routledge.

Berman, H. (2019). Redressing social injustice: Transcending and transforming the board of art therapy training in South Africa. In A. DiMaria (Ed.), *Exploring ethical dilemmas in art therapy, 50 clinicians from 20 countries share their stories* (pp. 68–75). Routledge.

Carliér, N., & Salom, A. (2012). When art therapy migrates: The acculturation challenge of sojourner art therapists. *Art Therapy: Journal of the American Art Therapy Association, 29*(1), 4–10. https://doi.org/10.1080/07421656.2012.648083

Chang, R. J. J. (2021). *Exploring Taiwanese creative arts therapists' professional identity after returning home from studying abroad.* Publication doctoral dissertation, Leslsy University.

Chong, F. H. H., & Liu, H. Y. (2002). Indigenous counseling in the Chinese cultural context: Experience transformed model. *Asian Journal of Counseling, 9*(1–2), 49–68.

Corey, G., Corey, M., & Corey, C. (2019). *Issues and ethics in the helping profession* (10th ed.). Cengage.

Donald, K. (2019). No man, or woman, is an island—Especially on an island: Practicing art therapy in the West Indies. In A. DiMaria (Ed.), *Exploring ethical dilemmas in art therapy, 50 clinicians from 20 countries share their stories* (pp. 111–117). Routledge.

Garlock, L. (2019). Art for sale? Using client art for promotional purposes. In A. DiMaria (Ed.), *Exploring ethical dilemmas in art therapy, 50 clinicians From 20 countries share their stories* (pp. 140–146). Routledge.

Hodges, J., & Oei, T. P. S. (2007). Would Confucius benefit from psychotherapy? The compatibility of cognitive behaviour therapy and Chinese values. *Behaviour Research and Therapy, 45*(5), 901–914. http://doi.org/10.1016/j.brat.2006.08.015

Huang, K. Y. (2021). Toward and indigenization process: Art therapy practice in the Chinese cultural context. *Art Therapy: Journal of the American Art Therapy Association.* http://doi.org/10.1080/07421656.2021.1919007

Hwang, K. K. (2009). The development of indigenous counseling in contemporary Confucian communities. *Counseling Psychologist*, *37*(7), 930–943. http://doi:10.1177/0011000009336241

Hwang, K. K. (2012). *Foundation of Chinese psychology: Confucian social relations.* Springer.

Hwang, W. C., Wood, J. J., Lin, K. M., & Cheung, F. (2006). Cognitive-behavioral therapy with Chinese Americans: Research, theory, and clinical practice. *Cognitive and Behavioral Practice*, *13*(4), 293–303. http://doi: 10.1016/j.cbpra.2006.04.010

Kalmanowitz, D., & Potash, J. S. (2010). Ethical considerations in the global teaching and promotion of art therapy to non-art therapists. *Arts in Psychotherapy*, *37*(1), 20–26. https://doi.org/10.1016/j.aip.2009.11.002

Keshri, V., & Garg, B. (2021). Operational barriers in providing comprehensive emergency obstetric care by task shifting of medical officers in selected states of India. *Indian Journal of Community Medicine*, *46*(2), 252–257. https://ww.doi.org/10.4103/ijcm.IJCM_563_20

Leenstra, S., Goldstraw, S., & Rumbold, B. (2014). Thinking about the arts as evidence. *Journal of Applied Arts and Health*, *5*(2), 227–234. https://doi-org.libezproxy2.syr.edu/10.1386/jaah.5.2.227_1

Leone, L. (Ed.). (2021). *Craft in art therapy: Diverse approaches to the transformative power of craft materials and methods.* Routledge.

Markus, H. R., & Kitayama, S. (1991). Culture and the self: Implications for cognition, emotion, and motivation. *Psychological Review*, *98*(2), 224–253. http://doi:10.1037/0033-295x.98.2.224

Martin, M. (2019). Art therapist. Yes! Minister. That too! Ethical issues that may arise when one has many roles. In A. DiMaria (Ed.), *Exploring ethical dilemmas in art therapy, 50 clinicians from 20 countries share their stories* (pp. 36–42). Routledge.

McNiff, S. (1997). Art therapy: A spectrum of partnerships. *The Arts in Psychotherapy*, *24*(1), 37–44. https://doi.org/10.1016/S0197-4556(97)00001-4

Moon, B., & Nolan, E. (2020). *Ethical issues in art therapy* (4th ed.). Charles C. Thomas.

Moon, C. H. (1997). Art therapy: Creating the space we will live in. *The Arts in Psychotherapy*, *24*(1), 45–49. https://doi.org/10.1016/S0197-4556(97)00003-8

Moon, C. H., & Shuman, V. (2013). The community art studio creating a space of solidarity and inclusion. In S. Prasad, P. Howie, & J. Kristel (Eds.), *Using art therapy with diverse populations: Crossing cultures and abilities* (pp. 297–307). Jessica Kingsley Publishers.

Morris, F. J., & Willis-Rauch, M. (2014). Join the art club: Exploring social empowerment in art therapy. *Art Therapy*, *31*(1), 28–36. https://doi.org/10.1080/07421656.2014.873694

Orkin, A., Rao, S., Venugopal, J., Kithulegoda, N., Wegier, P., Ritchie, S., VanderBurgh, D., Martiniuk, A., Salamanca-Buentello, F., & Upshur, R. (2021). Conceptual framework for task shifting and task sharing: An international Delphi study. *Human Resources for Health*, *19*(61), 1–8. https://doi.org/10.1186/s12960-021-00605-z

Osei, M. (2019). Hovering between art education and "art therapy'. In A. DiMaria (Ed.), *Exploring ethical dilemmas in art therapy, 50 clinicians from 20 countries share their stories* (pp. 204–209). Routledge.

Park, B. (2017). A Korean art therapist's autoethnography concerning re-acculturation to the motherland following training in the UK. *International Journal of Art Therapy*, *22*(4), 154–161. http://doi:10.1080/17454832.2017.1296008

Park, S. (2019). Translation of the therapeutic language: Can one teach or practice ethically without considering culture? In A. DiMaria (Ed.), *Exploring ethical dilemmas in art therapy: 50 clinicians from 20 countries share their stories* (pp. 76–82). Routledge.

Potash, J. (2019). Actually Hong Kong is a small town: Art therapy and multiple relationships in a community. In A. DiMaria (Ed.), *Exploring ethical dilemmas in art therapy: Clinicians from 20 countries share their stories* (pp. 191–196). Routledge.

Reyes, H. P. (2019). Art therapy in Chile: The ethical issues of an emerging professional practice. In A. DiMaria (Ed.), *Exploring ethical dilemmas in art therapy, 50 clinicians from 20 countries share their stories* (pp. 27–35). Routledge.

Shen, C. H. (2001). A study of counseling therapeutic factors for clients in material violence [in Chinese]. *Guidance Journal, 22*, 157–191.

Solomon, G. (2006). Development of art therapy in South Africa. *Canadian Art Therapy Association Journal, 19*(1), 17–32. http://doi:10.7040/GJ.200106.0157

Stoll, B. (2005). Growing pains: The international development of art therapy. *Arts in Psychotherapy, 32*(3), 171–191. https://doi.org/10.1016/j.aip.2005.03.003

Timm-Bottos, J. (1995). ArtStreet: Joining community through art. *Art Therapy, 12*(3), 184–187. https://doi.org/10.1080/07421656.1995.10759157

Vick, R. (2011). Ethics on exhibit. *Art Therapy, 28*(4), 152–158.

Vivian, J. (2019). Walking a new path: Indigenizing art therapy in Canada. In A. DiMaria (Ed.), *Exploring ethical dilemmas in art therapy, 50 clinicians from 20 countries share their stories* (pp. 83–88). Routledge.

Wolf Bordonaro, G. P. (2016). International art therapy. In M. Rosal & D. Gussak (Eds.), *Wiley Blackwell handbook of art therapy* (pp. 675–682). Wiley-Blackwell. https://doi.org/10.1002/9781118306543

Yang, K. S. (1995). Chinese social orientation: An integrative analysis. In T. Y. Lin, W. S. Tseng, & E. K. Yeh (Eds.), *Chinese societies and mental health* (pp. 19–39). Oxford University Press.

Chapter 6

Creating and Evaluating
Community Programs

Emily Goldstein Nolan and Rachel Monaco

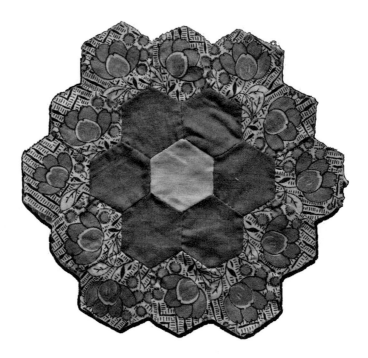

Honeycomb quilt block 6

The summer of 2016 was one of unrest in the city of Milwaukee. A young
Black man, Sylville Smith, was shot by the police and many protests followed.
One result of the turmoil left a bank in the Sherman Park neighborhood of the
city in embers. At that time, the community began to talk about what they could
do to build their neighborhood to be stronger and more resilient. In this case,
the transformation of the vestiges and what they build would consider the community's voice. Joanne Sabir and Juli Kaufman, together with the community,

DOI: 10.4324/9781003193289-6

opened the enterprise called Sherman Phoenix in 2019. Out of the ashes of the old, the Sherman Phoenix was born to foster desired and needed community change. It is a hub of primarily Black-owned businesses that brings together opportunities for the community to engage with food, wellness resources, and cultural activities. In 2020, developers invited Bloom to share space in the Sherman Phoenix to bring resonant services and its presence to the collective. Our reputation for meeting the community where they are, offered Bloom the opportunity to be in the Sherman Phoenix. Bloom held a location in the Sherman Phoenix from 2020 to 2023, where the organization operated as a member of that community, sharing resources, and amplifying the community's creative strengths.

What Happens With a Need and an Idea?

With the right relationships, planning, strategizing, acting, and reflecting, needs and ideas can become vibrant showcases of community. Not all ideas work, and careful planning, organizing, and networking can make the difference. In fact, my first attempt to create an art therapy program failed. Early on in my career, I thought that a local school in my neighborhood should offer art therapy, and with the help of an art therapy student I was supervising, we wrote a proposal and sent it to the school district. I never heard back from anyone at that district. Looking back on that experience now, we did not understand the unique needs of the school, lacked clear objectives for what we were offering, and had no relationships with the district leadership or local teachers. The approach I used to propose the program was not community-oriented, strategic, and my reflection now reveals insights as to why it failed.

Community programming that involves art therapy can occur in many ways and is only contained by the limits of collective dreaming. Programs might develop at their origin from the mind of an art therapist or collaborators may seek out art therapists as synergistic partners. However, I have seen that the most successful community programs including art therapy develop collectively, engaging stakeholders, and partners in community wellness from the very beginning.

Action Research and Program Development

Art therapists who wish to help create platforms for community art therapy can use an action research mindset to build them. Action researchers initiate program development by assessing the needs of the community, addressing gaps in available services, amplifying community strengths, and evaluating the effectiveness and sustainability of projects. Action research was initially developed by Kurt Lewin (1946) as a research model to "emphasize making an immediate difference in the world" (Willis & Edwards, 2014, p. 11.) Action research is a systematic form of investigation and "typically involves attempts to solve practical problems in real world settings through the involvement of stakeholders who work or live in those settings" (p. 19). Fals Borda also developed participatory action research methods that viewed knowledge as socially constructed and lived experience as best explored through group and social efforts (Robles Lomeli & Rappaport, 2018). In this chapter, action research is used as a mental framework or mindset for developing relevant community programming in a systematic way (see Figure 6.1) with continued opportunities for evaluation. If an art therapist wishes to write or publish work about their projects or thinks that they might want to do this later, then this would require an Institutional Review Board approval. Research is discussed further in Chapter 7.

Possible art therapy endeavors can be created and evolve through a cycle. First, community collaborators including the art therapist become aware of or attuned to a need. A passionate group of people gathers others to form a working group. The group determines some sense of shared leadership and member roles. Next, they develop the idea, or a collective vision, then test that idea against the needs of the community by gathering information. Once the idea for the program is developed and refined, it is implemented, observed, and evaluated, then further refined, thus beginning the cycle again (see Figure 6.2). Within the iterative cycles related to community art therapy program development are the

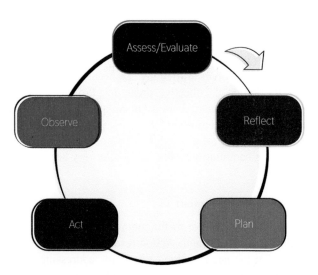

Figure 6.1 Action research cycle. General conceptualization of the action research cycle for program development and evaluation. The needs assessment takes place during the *assess/evaluate* portion of the cycle and a plan for program evaluation occurs at the outset

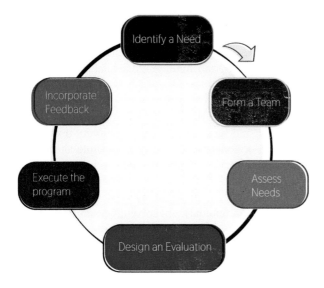

Figure 6.2 Program evolution. More specific representation of the process of program evolution from creation through incorporation of evaluative information

processes of 1) seeing/feeling/identifying a need, 2) forming a team to do the work and collaborate on the vision, 3) conducting a needs assessment to begin the process of planning, 4) designing a program evaluation to determine that the needs of the collective (which can be complex, including funders' goals, for example) and goals of the project have been met and illuminate outcomes, 5) executing the project/program or main steps of it, and 6) incorporating the evaluation feedback.

Once collaborators assemble and create the collective vision, the group conducts the needs assessment. The needs assessment considers several questions in gathering information to develop programming goals and implementation (Ritter & Lampkin, 2012).

Who is included when determining who will use this program?
How is the community defined and who is included in that community?
What do the community members identify as their wants/needs?
What is already being done to address the wants/needs?
What has been done previously to address wants/needs?
Were those ways effective or include aspects that were valuable?
How can art and aesthetic components address the wants/needs in a creative way that other avenues may not be able to impact?
What community growth or change can art influence?

How can the art provide advocacy?
What community strengths can be leveraged?
How does art play a role?
Are there any potential harms to the community or ethical challenges?
What resources, skills, services, goods, and funding are available and in what
    way?

The needs assessment compares what is currently happening to what is desired, defines the problem or concerns, and seeks to help the community understand what contributes to the problem or concerns. It also decides if the situation is dynamic, "determining if and how specific behaviors and mechanisms can be changed to produce the desired condition, developing solution strategies, and building support for action" (Sleezer et al., 2014). In my view, not all resources (including services, skills, goods, and funding) will solve the needs of the community, even if they are available.

The creativity in developing programs that involve art therapy lies in knowing how art therapy can contribute in some meaningful way. Once collaborators determine their vision for the program, it must align with what the community voices, which can be done through interviews, surveys, and focus groups. All of this considers general community concerns and what they wish to celebrate and amplify as community strengths. After collecting the relevant data, the collaborators engage in a filtering and sorting process to match resources to needs. Once the key players (WHO) and the vision, goals, and objectives (WHY) align with the resources of the community (HOW) and are in place, the project (WHAT) can start.

Evaluation

The action research process helps test what is happening in the program by engaging in cycles of action that collaborators can observe to determine the effects and impacts of those actions.

Once the project is underway, the community members carefully observe what happens next. The community observations help to refine how the program is implemented. Refinement includes changes in the how, the who, and, most importantly, sometimes even the "why" that has been chosen as a program goal. Evaluation can happen at any point, including after the last refined action or when new action has been implemented and observed.

Planning for evaluation can happen before program implementation to decide what to measure and how. In many cases, for funders to agree to provide the needed capital to move forward, early design is a must. At its best, program evaluation is systematic; it improves and accounts for community project effectiveness by collecting, analyzing, and sharing information regarding program goals and objectives. Through program evaluation, practitioners conduct systematic data collection and analysis to improve clinical and research practice, learn about patient perspectives, engage participants' voices in programming and planning, help generate evidence for funding opportunities, integrate arts-based program evaluation strategies, initiate research-related reflections, and document lessons learned.

(Kaimal & Blank, 2015, p. 89)

Kaimal and Blank (2015) distinguished the difference between program evaluation as evaluation and as research: evaluation is reactive while research is active. However, I see that art therapists and collaborators can use program evaluation as both, following proper institutional review; because what is learned from program evaluation can inform how programs continue to be implemented in the future, especially those that are replicated.

Programs get evaluated in two ways: through process evaluation and/or outcome evaluation (Kapitan, 2018). Process evaluation happens when program administrators, collaborators, and/or outside evaluators measure if the program is meeting needs while participants are engaged in the program, and if the program has been "delivered as intended" (Feldman et al., 2014, p. 102). For example, Bloom used process evaluation at the daytime shelter for people who are unhoused. Each semester the interns collected the number of unique individuals and counted how many sessions each person attended the community art therapy drop-in studio. Then Bloom provided the information back to the shelter to let them know that not only are people using the services but also there are a number of people who attend the studio regularly. Providing the numbers back to the shelter administration helped tie together the positive benefits that shelter staff may have observed with the shelter members because of the availability and use of art therapy. Providing the participation data back to the shelter kept the program relevant and anchored the collaboration between the shelter and Bloom in contributing to community healing.

Outcome Evaluation in a School Community

Outcome evaluation happens when program administrators, collaborators, and outside evaluators use data to show that a program is effective in what it purports to impact or change (Kapitan, 2018; Feldman et al., 2014). Bloom is a part of a restorative educational program in the Milwaukee Public Schools called the Success Center. The therapeutic program offers art therapy, dance/movement and drumming, and yoga in addition to traditional mental health therapy for students and their families. The program targets 4th- to 12th-grade students who would benefit from increased support to be successful in an academic setting. Students leave their school of origin to participate in the program for a period of nine weeks. Because current educational practices have been ingrained to demand student compliance, which is not effective for all students, faculty and staff work to create cultural change. The work empowers educators, therapists, and administrators to work from a restorative perspective.

A restorative model is key to the program rationale. This model uses many tools and much support to create an overall culture of care with the goal of interrupting the school-to-prison cycle for so many marginalized youth (Garnett et al. 2019; McCluskey et al., 2008; Selman et al., 2013; Wadha, 2016). The culture created at the Success Center is empathetic and the restorative model focuses on engaging in healthy relationships to prevent conflict and address behavioral concerns. The program uses transformational processes and interventions, or circles, to repair harm, help the student build success, and then transition back to their school of origin.

As the program has developed since 2019, the program administrators have provided process data to the district to show what is happening and ensure district support and sustainability. Now that the Success Center has had several cohorts of students move through the program, collaborators are refining what to use as data to show outcomes and how they collect the outcome data. So far, the program has collected reports from students, families, teachers, and school administration about how they see a child has benefited.

More specifically, a portfolio creation has become a primary evaluative method. The center has implemented a set of collective themes that students focus on in each therapeutic area during their nine weeks in the program. Each therapeutic partner gives the student a chance to focus on the weekly theme in their class. The center collects evidence of the students' meeting school, community, and individual goals using a portfolio that gathers evidence of the work the child has done in the program in each of the therapeutic areas attending to the collective theme for the week. The portfolios are used to show that the student has successfully moved through the program and can return to their home school. The center is working to ensure the successful transition back to the home school by building an infrastructure within the district to continue providing helpful services. In the future, the center will continue to monitor student progress through interviews, keeping track of grades, and discipline concerns after they have completed the program to collect longitudinal data. The center is still determining how to effectively evaluate community change because of the work happening within the program.

The Center for Disease Control and Prevention, or CDC offers a recommended six-step general framework for program evaluation in community health contexts (see Figure 6.3), (Centers for Disease Control and Prevention, 2017). The evaluation process put forth can be used in the action research cycle to gain both process and outcome data. The steps that the CDC provides are as follows:

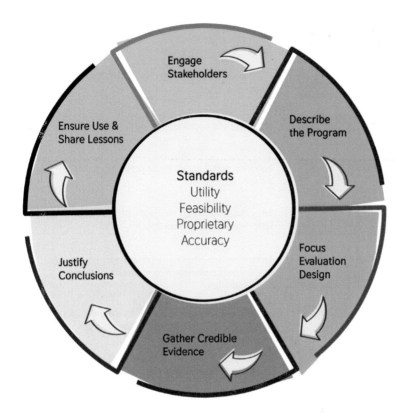

Figure 6.3 Program evaluation. Centers for Disease Control and Prevention. Framework for program evaluation in public health.

Credit: MMWR 1999;48 (No. RR-11) (2017)

Step 1: Engage community member stakeholders in the evaluation process.
Step 2: Provide a program description.
Step 3: Focus the evaluation design.
Step 4: Collect credible evidence.
Step 5: Validate the conclusions.
Step 6: Ensure use and communicate lessons learned.

One further source of insight to layer into evaluation addresses the role of the arts directly. Animating Democracy is a program through Americans for the Arts dedicated to civic engagement using art for social change (Animating Democracy, n.d.). The program has modeled a guiding set of aesthetics and values (Figure 6.4) for creating and evaluating community art programs. A layered

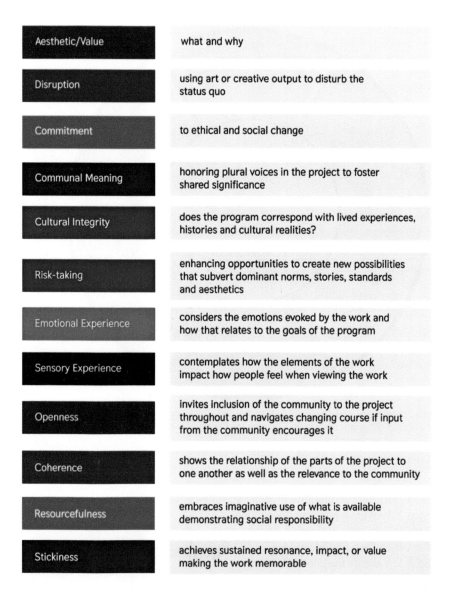

Aesthetic/Value	what and why
Disruption	using art or creative output to disturb the status quo
Commitment	to ethical and social change
Communal Meaning	honoring plural voices in the project to foster shared significance
Cultural Integrity	does the program correspond with lived experiences, histories and cultural realities?
Risk-taking	enhancing opportunities to create new possibilities that subvert dominant norms, stories, standards and aesthetics
Emotional Experience	considers the emotions evoked by the work and how that relates to the goals of the program
Sensory Experience	contemplates how the elements of the work impact how people feel when viewing the work
Openness	invites inclusion of the community to the project throughout and navigates changing course if input from the community encourages it
Coherence	shows the relationship of the parts of the project to one another as well as the relevance to the community
Resourcefulness	embraces imaginative use of what is available demonstrating social responsibility
Stickiness	achieves sustained resonance, impact, or value making the work memorable

Figure 6.4 Aesthetic attributes of creative change.

Credit: The authors' adaptation listing the aesthetic attributes of creative change (Borzel et. al., 2017)

approach makes sense: using the steps provided by the CDC while considering the aesthetics and values of Animating Democracy can be a meaningful way to design and engage in program evaluation.

Example of Program Evaluation

LOTUS Legal Clinic's Untold Stories Program serves as an example of how community art therapy became an essential part of meeting the needs of victims of sexual violence, using a humanities-based, restorative justice process to change the justice system and culture. LOTUS (Legal Options for Trafficked and Underserved Survivors) began in concept as a legal clinic at Mount Mary University when Rachel Monaco was Chair of the Justice Program. By 2016, LOTUS emerged as a freestanding nonprofit. The action research model, informed by the CDC steps and the aesthetic attributes from the Americans for the Arts programs, can illustrate how collaborators worked through the Untold Stories program's creation and growth alongside the development of LOTUS. Breaking each facet down with some explanation shows how Untold Stories evolved over its lifespan through the evaluation process and action research feedback loop.

In 2013, Rachel Monaco, JD, founder of LOTUS Legal Clinic, then professor of the Justice Program at Mount Mary University in Milwaukee, joined forces with the Voices and Faces Project to create the first Untold Stories program. The Voices and Faces Project delivered a weekend testimonial writing workshop called "The Stories We Tell"™ to applicants who identified as survivors of sexual violence. Testimonial writing focuses on,

> creating a community of activists ready to go public with their stories. The power of the stories emerging from The Stories We Tell is twofold. They call the public to an honest accounting of gender-based violence, and they attest to the strength that survivors find in a safe, creatively challenging community.
>
> (Voices and Faces Project, 2021)

The participants developed their written work with Rachel and English graduate writing-program faculty member Ann Angel over the next few months, and then shared it publicly through a Spring Showcase. The Spring Showcase promoted awareness, fueled advocacy, and elevated the voices of the survivors. In 2015, early efforts at incorporating artwork into the program process began, and, in 2016. Emily helped develop this to include a community art therapy component. Over time, LOTUS recruited other community partners including the Milwaukee Institute of Art and Design, and in 2019 LOTUS hired a full-time program director to bring Untold Stories fully under the nonprofit's Survivor Empowerment work. In its current form, Untold Stories is a year-round cycle that incorporates a writing workshop for survivors of sexual violence or exploitation, art therapy response art aimed at building empathy, a public showcase event for all participants and the community, a published magazine of the art and writing, and numerous other public exhibitions that arise throughout the year such as gallery nights, poetry readings, and legislative hearings.

The following describes how Rachel Monaco used the action research process and evaluative models for and within Untold Stories.

APPLYING THE ACTION RESEARCH CYCLE AND AESTHETIC ATTRIBUTES TO UNTOLD STORIES

Rachel Monaco

Identifying a Need

In 2013, while teaching and working in Milwaukee specifically with survivors of sexual violence and human trafficking, I (Rachel) began to see, and feel frustrated about, gaps and needs within the status quo. I saw that legal justice was either totally unavailable or missing the mark for most sexual violence survivors. Survivors wanted authentic ways to be true to their unique voices and experiences but lacked safe and effective means, skills, and venues. Worse, dominant narratives in the media did not come close to the diversity and nuance required to make better policy and create real culture change. I witnessed that there was a thirst for community among and between survivors and for caring spaces that did not further isolate or pathologize them. Finally, and most emotional for me, I saw that the brilliance and beauty of the individual survivors seeking some kind of creative outlet for their voice was undeniable. Their voices needed to be heard.

I assessed needs to gain feedback about who, what, why, how, where, and within what broader contexts Untold Stories needed to operate. With collaborators, I asked and listened to stakeholders that included:

- Student perspectives in classes such as Women, Crime, and Justice, and Abuse in the Justice System, a course in Mount Mary's Justice Program;
- Staff, administrators, and survivors in southeastern Wisconsin who worked with LOTUS Legal Clinic or with domestic violence shelters, homeless youth advocacy organizations, faith-based institutions;
- Lawyers, judges, attorneys, police, corrections staff, and health care workers who worked with sexual violence or its consequences on a regular basis.

In this case, I did not complete a formal needs assessment, and relied more organically upon collaborators and communication from key partners. With Untold Stories, there was an automatic synergy and overlap between the ongoing work of LOTUS in the community, the constant evaluation of its own methods, the needs of the community, and the change LOTUS sought to create with its programs. We continually assessed needs at every staff meeting, every board meeting, and in the writing of every grant report (see Figure 6.5).

Forming a Team to Do the Work and Collaborate on the Vision

In 2013, my initial vision for Untold Stories invited the Voices and Faces Project to provide the writing workshop component for the survivors. I applied for grants: our major funder was the Wisconsin Humanities Council. I had a supportive Justice Advisory Board through my position at Mount Mary University, which served as a collaborative sounding board for the development of Untold Stories in the early years. Over time, different key

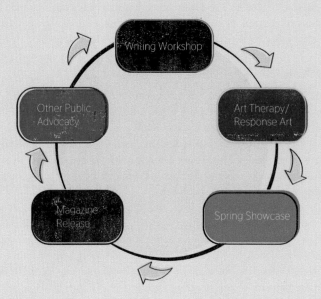

Figure 6.5 The year-round cycle of the Untold Stories program of LOTUS Legal Clinic in 2019

volunteers from the community played a role. In 2015, I forged new alliances with the nonprofit Arts @ Large and Bloom Art and Integrated Therapies, Inc. Through Arts @ Large and Bloom, the written work of the survivors was brought to area middle school and high school students with the goal of building empathy through responding to the survivor's written work through artmaking.

In 2016, LOTUS got its nonprofit status. In 2017, I left Mount Mary to run LOTUS full time, and brought Untold Stories under LOTUS's Survivor Empowerment branch. From the beginning, together with my collaborators, I planned each year's approach in the quiet months in between the Spring Showcase and the next year's fall writing workshop. Through reflection in action, I observed a need for changes. One of the first changes was to collaborative partnerships; for example, the community and participant feedback from the Spring Showcase one year made it clear that the program had risen to a new level of public scrutiny and potential policy impact on victim's law. The advisory board wondered what it would be like to have different artists respond to the survivor's written work. With that feedback in mind, Untold Stories formed an alliance with Milwaukee Institute of Art and Design. The new action informed by the action research cycle was choosing to have the response art created by an older and more experienced group of artists rather than working with junior high and high school students.

Designing a Program Evaluation

Because Untold Stories was grant dependent, I got in the habit early on of coming up with ways to measure impact. Fortunately, the main funder, the Wisconsin Humanities Council, was brilliant in giving the Untold Stories team the freedom to creatively assess and evaluate what happened. They communicated that making mistakes and learning from them (process evaluation) was as important as meeting anticipated numeric or qualitative (outcomes) goals that were set prior to each year.

My team and I used short-, mid-, and long-term survey processes at each stage of the program cycle (writing workshop, art making by students, Spring Showcase). These were sometimes paper surveys, survey monkeys, gathering unsolicited feedback, holding focus groups, and having one-on-one mentoring conversations. The use of many layers of evaluation was possible because former participants of the program kept in touch. The participants formed strong social (and sometimes legal, through LOTUS work and legal representation) bonds with the program director, LOTUS staff, volunteers, and each other. The feedback from participants helped inform our formal evaluation processes. Depending on the population and the issues of the work, it may not always be necessary, appropriate, ethical, or helpful to use an overly for-mulaic evaluation tool. Listening to each individual voice with respect and in safety should anchor all processes. The narratives the participants give about the benefits of participation are invaluable.

Survivors who took part in future public or advocacy efforts on their own initiative as program alums provided much evaluative data. For example, when an alum published her first book, a memoir about two teen Latinx women and their overcoming sexual abuse, she tied her journey back to her experience in Untold Stories as a catalyst.

Executing the Project

The program evolved in this phase because collaborators and I learned as we went. I was open to possibility through development but always prioritized the main vision of the program. It was important to honor the relationships with the collaborators while facing resource needs, availability of spaces, transportation for participants, accessibility needs (the food! the stairs! the party on floor 2 of the building!) funds, materials, time and energy, and work-ing through challenges (something will always go haywire).

Incorporating the Feedback Into the Next Cycle

In the pauses between each segment of the Untold Stories program, I inte-grated changes: 1) I reviewed the feedback collected and reflected on the synergy with LOTUS's mission and strategic vision since I held both roles of Untold Stories program director and LOTUS CEO until 2019; 2) I wrote post-event reports throughout the year and shared with the staff and board; 3) I held team meetings with the collaborative partners; 4) I created the mar-keting and communications for Untold Stories and LOTUS, and wrote grant reports due on a schedule to our funders and finally; 5) I wrote the grant applications and told the story of the program, its people, work and impact for various reasons in each successive year when building up for the next cycle. I found that in today's competitive funding culture, making the case for what the program did and how it changed over time is not a choice—it's the only way to get sustainable support (see Figure 6.6).

Aesthetics and Values for Creating and Evaluating Community Art Programs

The Americans for the Arts provides a visual model (see Figure 6.7) that helps illustrate how all the aesthetics are in play from the creation of a program

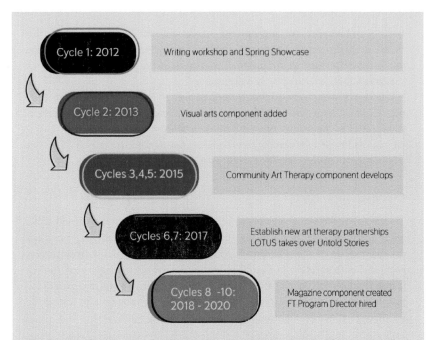

Figure 6.6 The evolution of Untold Stories over time, using the action research process, evaluation, and program development cycles

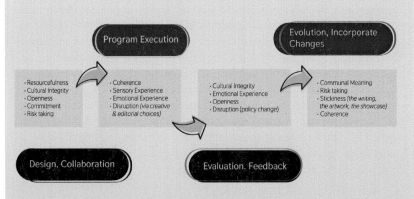

Figure 6.7 Aesthetics as applied to the program creation, execution, evaluation, and evolution process of Untold Stories

throughout delivery, evaluation, and incorporation of changes for evolution. Certain aesthetics were sometimes more active in the beginning stages of Untold Stories; other aesthetics had more power, influence, and were "louder" in the later phases of the program.

As the program matured over each successive year, some aesthetics needed more attention or increased in priority of focus, depending on how the cultural, social, and political context resonated with our program and its participants. For example, the rise of the MeToo movement in 2017 (Me Too, 2021) and Times Up™ in 2018 (Times Up, 2021) heightened survivors' feelings of vulnerability, shame, and ambivalence about needing to disclose publicly. The movements brought conversations about sexual violence out of safer spaces such as the workshop and into very public spaces such as social media where there was little to no control over how people responded to survivor testimony. This cultural backdrop required me to pay extra attention in Untold Stories to the aesthetics of risk-taking, emotional experience, sensory experience (PTSD symptoms being more easily triggered), cultural integrity (over the exclusion of non-white, higher socioeconomic status female voices). I had to weigh these with the benefits of the obvious focus on disruption, potential stickiness, communal meaning, and policy change that represented the aesthetics most resonant with those advocacy movements. I learned that not all forms of advocacy (protest marches, or engaging in social media opinion battles, for example) are beneficial in the short or long run for some survivors. Ensuring individual strategy, autonomy and choice in advocacy is a trauma-informed approach. Having the set of aesthetics as anchors to the evaluation of the program helped me narrate Untold Stories' methods *and* the impact to ourselves, our participants, our funders, and the community.

In hindsight, I see clearly how action research and evaluation generated significant and powerful changes for Untold Stories over a relatively short period of time. Writing this reflection helped me understand how some of the uncertainty, frustration, and doubt I felt at times as a leader during many of these cycles of change was normal, healthy, and important. My hope is that by seeing how the models operate for Untold Stories, the reader will be able to find footing in the process of constant adaptation and embrace it for the gift it delivers, confident that your work is making a difference.

Conclusion

Action research is used to implement change. In community, it is used as a participatory method to implement and develop new programs. The framework of action research allows communities and stakeholders opportunities to determine relevant needs as well as evaluate the effectiveness of what transpires to meet those needs. Art therapists are no strangers to the act of creation and engaging in the collaborative partnership of the creative process. Art therapists have unique skills that make them valuable to their communities and art therapy can contribute to new paths for societal change.

Art experience

Individual:

1. Create an image of what is happening in your community and what is needed. How might the community attend to that need?
2. Create an image of, and reflect on, a program that you tried to implement but failed. What was missing in the design and planning? What did you learn?

Community:

1. Create a collective image, or vision board of the most important things to consider when working together to create your efforts.
2. Create a collective image, or vision board of the most important things to consider when working together to evaluate your efforts.
3. Use these images to set a visual collective intention for both program development and evaluation.

References

Animating Democracy. (n.d.) A program of Americans for the arts. http://animatingdemocracy.org/

Borstel, J., Korza, P., Assaf, A., Dwyer, C., Valdez, C., and Brown, D. (2017, May 16). Aesthetic perspectives: Attributes of excellence in arts for change. Americans for the Arts. https://www.americansforthearts.org/sites/default/files/Aesthetic%20Perspectives%20Full%20Framework.pdf

Centers for Disease Control and Prevention. (1999). Framework for program evaluation in public health. *Morbidity and Mortality Weekly Report 1999, 48* (No. RR-11), 1–40.

Centers for Disease Control and Prevention. (2017). Framework for program evaluation in public health. https://www.cdc.gov/eval/framework/index.htm

Feldman, M., Betts, D., & Blausey, D. (2014). Process and outcome evaluation of an art therapy program for people living with HIV/AIDS. *Art Therapy*, *31*(3), 102–109. https://doi.org/10.1080/07421656.2014.935593

Garnett, B., Smith, L., Kervick, C., Ballysingh, T., Moore, M., & Gonell, E. (2019). The emancipatory potential of transformative mixed methods designs: Informing youth participatory action research and restorative practices within a district-wide school transformation project. *International Journal of Research and Method in Education*, *42*(3), 305–316. https://doi.org/10.1080/1743727X.2019.1598355

Kaimal, G., & Blank, C. (2015). Program evaluation: A doorway to research in the creative arts. *Art Therapy*, *32*(2), 89–92. https://doi.org/10.1080/07421656.2015.1028310

Kapitan, K. (2018). *Introduction to art therapy research* (2nd ed.). Routledge.

Lewin, K. (1946). Action research and minority problems. *Journal of Social Issues*, *2*(4), 34–46.

McCluskey, G., Lloyd, G., Stead, J., Kane, J., Riddell, S., & Weedon, E. (2008). 'I was dead restorative today': From restorative justice to restorative approaches in school. *Cambridge Journal of Education*, *38*(2), 199–216. https://doi.org/10.1080/03057640802063262

Me Too. (2021). https://metoomvmt.org/

Ritter, L., & Lampkin, S. (2012). *Community mental health*. Jones and Barlett learning.

Robles Lomeli, J. D., & Rappaport, J. (2018). Imagining Latin American social science from the global South: Orlando Fals Borda and participatory action research. *Latin American Research Review*, *53*(3), 597–612. http://doi.org/10.25222/larr.164

Sellman, E., Cremin, H., & McCluskey, G. (Eds.). (2013). *Restorative approaches to conflict in schools: Interdisciplinary perspectives on whole school approaches to managing relationships*. Routledge.

Sleezer, C., Russ-Eft, D., & Gupta, K. (2014). *A practical guide to needs assessment* (3rd ed.). Pfeiffer.

Times Up. (2021). https://timesupnow.org/

Voices and Faces Project. (2021). The stories we tell. https://voicesandfaces.org/workshop/.

Wadha, A. (2016). *Restorative justice in urban schools: Disrupting the school-to-prison pipeline*. Routledge.

Willis, J., & Edwards, C. (Eds.). (2014). *Action research: Models, methods, and examples*. Information Age Publishing.

Chapter 7

Research and Community

Rochele Royster and Emily Goldstein Nolan

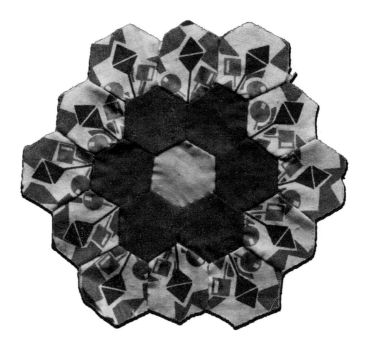

Honeycomb quilt block 7

Introduction

Grounding Research in Embodiment

At the start of this chapter, it is important to point out that research feels meaningful when it is connected, and in my experience of doing, participating in, and teaching research it often feels disconnected in many ways. Graduate art therapy students often report that research feels daunting and that it is difficult

DOI: 10.4324/9781003193289-7

to manage feelings of needing to master both practitioner and researcher skills while in graduate school (Abrams & Nolan, 2016). Both Kapitan (2018) and Leavy (2020) have noted the challenges of conducting research, in as far as feeling intimidated or as if the results are inaccurate portrayals of lived experience. I (Emily) often felt a disconnection between research and practice until I got my doctorate, where I learned that research is another form of my own creativity and that it informs practice and practice informs research. Until that time, I had this notion that research happened somewhere up high, divorced from any practical application. A part of that disconnection I see now as being and feeling disembodied.

Somatic therapies use the body as one more dimension of processing information in therapy; developing awareness of behavior, affect, and cognition are used in healing and transformation, as is attuning to somatic awareness. As a Somatic Experiencing® Practitioner, I have attended trainings on embodied research mentorship. Embodied researchers encourage people to use somatic methods in the process of research to ground one another and the work. Once I was able to connect research to my body of practice, and feel fully present and engaged doing it, I was able to participate in research with more intentionality and regulation.

Embodied research encourages awareness of how one shows up to do research. People experience the world and other through their bodies (Johnson, 2018). People learn from one another; grounded research embraces interdependence and mutuality. Grounded researchers actively seek out what is different from their perspective and are willing to be challenged; they meet others where they are with invitation and acceptance. The research process requires openness without holding onto preconceptions and lets the process unfold. Finally, ample time and space are taken to reduce overwhelm and allow for integration of insights. At the outset, this chapter encourages practitioners to develop and use somatic understandings of themselves and others while engaging in research and to consider best practices when researching in community art therapy contexts.

Social Research = Social Change

Practice-based research methods are qualitative and focused on relevance to how art therapy is conducted. At their root, qualitative research methods are constructivist, meaning that they are influenced by people's histories, cultures, and worldviews (Kapitan, 2018). The social world is constructed through people's interactions with others. Community art therapy is social, and therefore effective investigation can be done using qualitative research. Additionally, community art therapy relies on creativity and application of artistic endeavors in the social realm. Art can inform research in communities as well as include arts-based methods (Leavy, 2020).

Critical and social art therapy research, much like critical psychology and community psychology research is directly influenced by values and oriented toward social change (Prilleltensky & Nelson, 2002). Social change occurs using what is learned from research and implemented in practice. The goal of critical and social art therapy research is to positively change people, processes, and practice environments, which then in turn ripples out into the world, effectuating more change. "The use of research for systemic advocacy is critical for eradicating oppressive social structures and for promoting collective empowerment" (Prilleltensky & Nelson, 2002, p. 60). Involving communities in research, evolving practices with the people who are engaged in those practices only makes the services art therapists provide more meaningful.

From an anti-oppressive standpoint that actively includes communities in developing knowledge art therapists ask: Who benefits from the research, and how is the knowledge used? (Kapitan, 2018). Communities are involved and encouraged to become co-researchers following a Frierean underpinning of doing research *with* not *for* (Friere, 2012). When communities are involved and included, the research is participatory. Participatory "approaches provide the opportunities for communities to codevelop and thus allow for holistic self-determined interventions that reflect the life experiences, values, and goals of the community" (Oetzel et al., 2018, p. 11). Research shows that participatory research within communities builds capacity, and transforms communities and their health outcomes through the process and outcomes of the research.

However, critique of participatory research has questioned what it encompasses and what is truly meant by participation (Juan, 2021). The questioning asks whose voices are included and posits that well-meaning organizations can continue to reenact unequal power dynamics and impede transformation. My recommendation is to evaluate power dynamics and participation at each stage of a research project from pre-planning to post-research debriefing; requiring the researchers to continually ask who is included and how at each stage.

Challenges

Empowering the community in research is certainly a primary concern. However, I have seen challenges in conducting community research include the need to seed researchers' power when appropriate in oppressive systems. Navigating the Institutional Review Board process presents a challenge, at times, to explain the nuances of emergent qualitative, arts-based, and/or participatory research methods.

Research in community art therapy endeavors takes much longer than other research processes and this can be difficult. Researchers take time to develop relationships with stakeholders and engage in collaborative processes to ensure that power is shared. Data is often emergent and requires careful observation and analysis. Community art therapy researchers slow down to meet the process where it is, immersed in the richness of the process and the outcomes.

Research, in general, is often written in language that is academic—inaccessible or uninteresting. I often wonder how as an academic I can share my work in ways that are recognized as creative, scholarly, engaging, and available. One thing I have learned is that if I frame my sharing information and writing as storytelling, then it feels more alive and engaging to me.

In the following section, Rochele Royster provides a perspective on community art therapy research using the metaphor of salt. I find her writing on research accessible, inspiring, and hopeful.

SALT OF THE EARTH: RESEARCH AS PRAXIS

Rochele Royster

Salt as Metaphor

Research, like salt, is essential to life. It has pushed humanity forward, like our cultivation and comedication of salt that has helped us survive and flourish, but also has catalyzed systems of revolution, oppression, and war connecting us through time, space, and place. Bodies are born from salty waters; our tears and sweat reflect the same makeup of sodium and chloride found in the ocean. Humans become researchers at birth, fueled by natural curiosity, babies search for meaning in faces and sounds, children naturally ask questions, and adolescents test boundaries and social norms, immersing themselves in the process of knowledge and discovery. When I say "salt of the earth," the implication is great and encompasses all that is good, honest, and well in the world. Salt is a rich metaphor used in our history and language to narrate images of morality, judgment, death, and discipleship. My grandmother characterized the most honest, good, and hardworking people as "the salt of the earth." Let's dive into this metaphor and examine research in this way. If research *was the salt of the earth,* what would it be? How would it look?

Praxis

Application of research, theory, and action creates praxis. Praxis uses research and theory to initiate social action and create social change. Being curious and wanting to gain insight and knowledge while engaging in theoretical readings and discussions is imperative without negating practice for the sake of theory (Freire, 2012). Unity and balance between theory, practice, and reflection shapes praxis, which embodies certain qualities, ethics, and intentions. These qualities are an intentional commitment to the well-being of the individual, community, the earth, our search for truth, and respect for others. It is for the people, by the people, and liberatory in practice, theory, and action. In praxis-oriented research the community is involved in the research process and the researcher is doing research *with* the community, not *on* the community. Praxis can be rigorous, risky, and is consistently ever-changing. Praxis requires a researcher to constantly reflect, adjust, and use nonbiased judgment guided by a moral disposition to act with truth and a concern to further human and ecological well-being in any given situation. Critical reflection requires an understanding of people and human diversity in context to culture, race, ethnicity, age, spirituality, social class, ability/disability, age, sexual orientation, and the intersectionality of these systems. Practitioners question: What is the historical perspective of a community or society? How was it constructed and how is it sustained? What are the social determinants and context of the community in which I am involved in? Whose interests are served by current theory and research? (Kloos et al., 2012). Very naturally, sentient beings transform lived experiences into knowledge and use the acquired knowledge to process new knowledge.

> [Research] is the salt of the earth, but if the salt has lost its flavor, with what will it be salted? It is then good for nothing, but to be cast out and to be trodden under foot of men.
>
> Jesus (Matthew 5:13, King James Bible, 1769/2017)

Swampscott Conference 1965

In 1965, 39 individuals attended a conference in Swampscott, Massachusetts; frustrated, angered, and disappointed with the field of psychology and the mental health profession, they gathered to critique, imagine, and redefine how psychologists could become "change agents" and impact social change and policy beyond psychological therapeutic interventions (Bennett et al., 1966). It was not long before the climate of the conference became heated and ignited a flame. Conference attendees demanded a shift in perspective in psychology. Their observations and reflections on the field and current practices revealed the "old way" of doing things was not working and had been rooted in archaic ways of practicing that focused on intervention and disease, misogyny, racism, and classist practices. The Swampscott Conference was the container that held the liquid, as the agitators brought the liquid to boiling point.

The 1960s were turbulent times, defined by marches, movements, assassinations, and demonstrations sparked by several political and social change movements such as the Civil Rights Movement, Vietnam War, the feminist movement, and the Black Panther Party to name a few. It was also a time of deinstitutionalization of mental institutions, as images of horrible conditions in mental hospitals and the harmful effects of mental hospitalization were being revealed by the media (Erikson, 2021). The report of the Joint Commission on Mental Health and Illness was released in 1961 and recommended reducing the size of mental institutions and increasing opportunities for educating and training more professionals to meet the needs of the community through mental health services (Erikson, 2021). From the Swampscott Conference, community psychology was born, demanding a shift in perspective within psychology focusing on how an individual exists within a web of contexts, environments, and social connections (Kloos et al., 2012). Community psychology emerged in response to the limitations of psychology in solving social problems and was stimulated by the community mental health movement. The participants imagined an innovative approach to research and practice and pushed for an action-oriented psychology that emphasized education for prevention, innovative field training experiences, and the need to gain knowledge about communities through research and evaluation.

The de-institutionalization of psychiatric hospitals initiated a shift from long-term care to short-term care, an increase in community mental health centers and private hospitals and subsequently decreasing inpatient hospital care resulted in more homelessness and incarceration (Wallace, 2014). During this time, art therapists, Cliff Joseph and Georgette Seabrook Powell responded to this shift in care by creating more opportunities for structured and non-structured group therapy in the form of open art studios and collaborative murals to meet the community's mental health needs within schools, health centers, and psychiatric hospitals (Cliff, 2006; Black Smith, 2014; Stepney, 2019). Art was recognized as a tool to be used within treatment to facilitate growth and change of the individual and the community (Rubin, 2015).

Art-Based Research in Community

Art-based research (ABR) is an approach to knowledge-building involving inquiry, artmaking in various art forms, and is informed by the belief that combining arts and humanities can facilitate scientific goals. Researchers intentionally engage in artmaking as a way of knowing and understanding the self and our relationship to others in the built world (McNiff, 2013). ABR embodies multiple ways of knowing, transcending language and interlocking the body and mind in new discoveries. Art-based research can offer new insights and learning, make connections, ask, and answer questions and represent research and data visually (Leavy, 2020).

ABR can be used to raise consciousness and empathy, reveal power dynamics, and challenge stereotypes. It can heighten and amplify the voices of the community. The use of ABR with community can level the playing field, allowing participants and researchers to be equal participants and learners in the process of discovery.

Salt of the Earth: Community Psychology Frameworks and Principles Applied to Art Therapy

Shift in Perspective (Ecological/ Empirical Research)

A community psychology framework demands a shift in thinking and adopts an ecological perspective which pushes the boundaries of psychology beyond an individualistic perspective to consider how individuals, families, communities, and societies are interconnected and impacted by local and national policies and governance (Jason et al., 2019, para 8). The environment plays a critical part when trying to understand and work with communities and the individuals in them. Salt-of-the-earth research considers multiple ecological levels of communities:

- How are communities defined?
- Who has defined the community?
- Is there a counternarrative?

Communities offer rich opportunities for research, integrating knowledge with action to pursue answers to questions about how communities shape their world and how their worlds shape them. What is the relationship between the individual and their environment? The act of observing and experimenting and then collecting the data from observable events is empirically grounded research. It integrates research with community action, using research to make community organizing more effective and transparent. Empirically grounded research is theory and scientific methods proven effective using quantitative and qualitative research methods (Kloos et al., 2012).

Research as Social Justice

Social justice as a term and definition is often used broadly but can be refined further, highlighting the juxtaposition of process and product, procedure, and outcome, in the distribution of democracy. Social justice is the "equitable allocation of resources, opportunities, and power in society" (Prilleltensky, 2001, p. 754). How are resources distributed and who determines how the resources are distributed? A social justice perspective is concerned with advocacy for social change. This perspective shows concern for wellness, citizenship, inclusion, and diversity. Research aimed at changing social practices and processes for the betterment of the community is justice-oriented (Johnson, 2014).

Research is Prevention

Research can be preventative and foster social change. With a focus on prevention in communities versus *intervention*, or reactionary practices, research is strength-based and works to build the positive attributes of a community. Amplifying strengths promotes resilience and recovery when tragic or traumatic events happen. Preventative programs act as a safety net for the community to ensure repair and resilience after a crisis.

Research is Reflexive

Researchers strive to be reflexive by stating their interests, values, preconceptions, and personal statuses or roles as explicitly as possible to all participants including research participants and researchers. This supports transparency, lessens bias and assumptions, and invites participants to control and contribute to how they are reflected and represented in the disseminated research.

Research is Collaborative and Shares Power

Interventions, preventative program design, and research are a collaborative effort. Working across dimensions breaks down power dynamics that can easily be formed when a researcher, who is often viewed as the expert, works within the community. Using a collaborative model of research provides vital information from many different perspectives, encouraging critical inquiry and dialogue which may lead to a successful and meaningful project.

Research Shows Cultural Humility

Diversity is respected and represented in salt-of-the-earth research. Individuals function through cultural and social contexts and achieve a sense of community with diverse environments. No person is an expert on every dimension of diversity and the human experience. Although cultural competence encompasses respect for others and a realization of one's own biases, cultural humility is an active practice that requires a constant critical gaze on his, her or their personal limitations, racist assumptions, and anti-Blackness that is embedded in every aspect of our lives, such as social media, public policy, education, and the overall dogma upheld and reinforced by white supremacy. Cultural humility offers understanding about how humans differ across cultural, racial, ethnic, gender and other boundaries as well as our commonalities and begins with a thorough examination of one's personal beliefs, familial upbringing, and cultural identities (Jackson, 2020).

Research Values a Sense of Community

A sense of community is interdependence on others and the feeling that one is part of a larger structure that is dependable and stable (Sarason, 1988). Community requires that people feel a sense of belonging and a shared understanding that the needs of the members will be met through their commitment to each other together. The use of mutual aid offers community care focused on the greater good. Mutual aid is the radical act of caring for each other while working to mobilize, transform and activate communities despite obstacles, oppression, and discrimination (Spade 2020). Mutual aid in community art therapy is "holding space and holding change" (Brown, 2021); nurturing, cultivating, and harvesting change at the individual and collective level through intentional creative art actions as a form of resistance to the status quo.

Research Empowers Citizen Participation

Empowerment is having access to valued resources and gaining true power and not just the feeling of being in control of one's life decisions (Zimmerman, 2000). Empowerment can involve collective action and decision-making such as citizen participation. Citizen participation is a process in which individuals take part in decision-making in the institutions, programs, and environments that affect them (Kloos et al., 2012); making the community member's voices heard and inviting them to influence decisions in democratic ways. Community arts research can amplify the collective voice of the community, bringing to light concerns, imagining, and offering solutions to create social change. An art action and the product (murals, installations, exhibits, photovoice, etc.) offers a visual experience to the problem in a creative and non-threatening way, shifting the perspective and influencing decisions in collective ways.

Research Supports Effective Coping Strategies

A salt-of-the-earth researcher seeks to improve community coping outcomes and reduce exposure to risk factors. Some stressors stretch beyond the individual and are often rooted in organizational and systemic conditions that require collective action.

Figure 7.1 shows key ingredients that create salt-of-the-earth research as praxis. The first ingredient, salt, is the question, phenomenon, or situation that is guiding the research. This is rooted in social justice and advocacy. Earth is the practical wisdom that is embodied by the researcher, community stakeholders and participants. It is honest community care and mutual aid. Praxis, research, theory, and action enable authentic engagement between self-aware and culturally humble and curious researchers and participants operating on equal planes. The interaction is the artwork, exhibition, and/or art action that is the outcome of the continuous process of community engagement and reflection. This circle is fueled by intention and motivation for the greater good and overall well-being of the community. The researcher and art therapist holds the space and change initially but intentionally works to create opportunities and experiences to build advocacy skills that are sustainable for community members after the research is completed.

Art Therapy as Prevention

I created a school-based after-school and summer art therapy program for teens promoting social emotional competence and civic engagement. This program (see Figure 7.1) provided teens with necessary coping skills, community support, and social emotional intelligence through psychoeducational outreach and art therapy community projects aimed at solving schoolwide and community problems. Students worked together to find solutions to problems through community engagement, communal artmaking, and public art actions. One problem was the entry hall to the cafeteria. This hallway was dark, neglected, and institutional. Parts of the wall had big holes where students continued to kick the plaster off the wall, the paint was old and dirty, and students enjoyed vandalizing the wall as they waited to enter the lunchroom. Data collected from the school's behavioral monitoring system indicated that fights would break out along this route as students waited to enter. The after-school program wanted to upgrade this eyesore and change the feeling of the hallway by painting murals along the walls. They incorporated students from all different grades so that the students felt ownership over the area. If students felt pride in their work, they would not want to

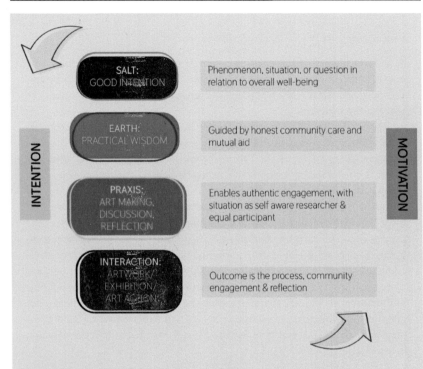

Figure 7.1 Salt-of-the-earth research as praxis

destroy it, or see others destroy it. The murals were created and selected by the school community, and every student participated in their selection, design, or creation. Students that had vandalized the wall or were chronic offenders in disrupting the area were especially targeted to help in the beautification efforts and some were made leaders in the project. The vandalism immediately stopped, fights decreased, and the hallway became a source of pride for the school community. This program is an example of preventative arts-based care supported by research. Preventative measures are important to protect physical health and imperative for mental and social health. If trauma or tragedy happens, individuals have effective coping strategies, practice in resilience, and an established supportive community as a safety net.

Art Therapy as Intervention and Advocacy

After the tragic shooting of a popular student within a small school community, I implemented an art intervention that invited students to grieve the death of the student and others who had been killed by gun violence that year. To process their feelings, I taught students to make simple wrap dolls out of craft and found objects such as fabric, string, yarn, feathers, and buttons. Students sat in maker circles creating dolls for loved ones who had died from gun violence while processing their thoughts and emotions. Students were holding space for each other using the art process as the impetus for their protest and creative resistance (Royster, 2021). Students shifted the focus from therapeutic intervention to sustainable community advocacy by facilitating maker circles in their own communal spaces. I was able to carry the research forward with the help of civic engaged cultural institutions, academic validation, grants from local art stores, and the support of educators who felt a visceral connection to the project. Educators also experienced their own losses and the collective trauma of witnessing the phenomenon of multiple school shootings and individual gun violence within the community. Students, community members, and I as researcher created a living memorial for those who had been shot and killed by gun violence; 56 schools, 6 colleges, and over 1,400 people made a doll for each person shot. The memorial was included in an exhibit at a popular cultural center/museum and people were invited to the memorial as a call to action. This call to action demanded more community art opportunities, after-school art and music programs, mental health access for teens, youth, and community members, and a trauma center in the community. The living memorial supported survivors by helping them heal and address community trauma caused by gun violence and brought attention to how this violence was impacting our homes, schools, and bodies. The community engaged the institutional structures and political figures by requesting a trauma center be rebuilt where one had been but had closed years earlier. The absence of the trauma center meant that gunshot victims in the area would have to be transported to a different part of the city which increased fatalities. This community action brought about change and empowered participants to initiate community change for the overall well-being of all.

In this example, the research process follows Figure 7.1.

Salt: Tragic shooting and the larger phenomenon of gun violence.
Earth: Art therapy intervention (doll-making and maker circles to process difficult feelings).
Praxis: The theory, research, and action that included the therapeutic maker circles, ongoing discussion, and reflection of the participants, stake holders, and researcher.
Interaction: The living memorial engaged community to reflect on needs, community strengths, and demand action.
Intention: To facilitate healing and awareness through sustainable student led maker spaces.

Motivation: Call to action for more mental health services, a trauma center, and the funding of art programs.

Salt of the Earth: Liberatory Practices in Research

> The revolutionary sees his task as liberation not only of the oppressed but also of the oppressor. Happiness can never truly exist in a state of tension.
>
> Steven Biko

When research is flavored as the salt of the earth, the result can enhance, preserve, fertilize, and/or destroy. The researcher is mindful of the people, places, practices, and tools included in the planning, process, and evaluation, always aware of their moral compass, and what the implications of the research will be for the community.

To Flavor

Salt enhances the flavors of the foods we eat. Community art therapy research enhances the community, makes it better by focusing on the strengths in the community, building opportunities for positive engagement, interactions, further establishing authentic connections and relations.

To Preserve

As salt is used to preserve, so should community art therapy research. Storytelling used in research keeps the lived experiences of people alive. Storytelling currently is an emergent research method or a circular process of data collection, procedural analysis, and reflection that evolves and changes with the project. Not fully validated by academia, storytelling should not be dismissed; it is important to, and prevalence in, Indigenous and African-centered cultures and ancient folklore and can be used as a tool to sustain intangible cultural heritage; it is an intentional act of documenting and safeguarding the process of cultural expression. Community art therapy research should be used as a tool and vehicle for amplifying the voice of the community by inviting the community to self-define, discover, and transform their own stories.

To Fertilize

Ancient civilizations used salt as fertilizer for the soil to make the fields easier to plow, release minerals, and stimulate growth. Research fertilizes our communities where conditions are challenging and hard. Research enriches, protects against disease, stimulates growth, and scatters sustainable change. Participants involved in research are equal partners and have access to the data but also to the universities in which art therapists work. Research is not a one-way street. The researcher is offered access to the inside workings of a community, and the community gets access to the institution the researcher represents.

To Destroy

Too much salt can wreak havoc. Heavy-handed research that does not examine and consider power dynamics can oppress, discriminate against, placate, or further marginalize communities. Art therapists use salt in the right proportions to do no harm.

Summary

Salt-of-the-earth praxis brings about a thirst for authentic research that is liberatory and transparent for the greater good of the community. It embraces change and centers that "small is all," a belief that the small will be reflected by the whole (Brown, 2021). Like the psychologists at the Swampscott Conference that demanded new ways of practice, researchers must reimagine ways of doing research that is anti-racist, non-oppressive, and community centered. Salt-of-the-earth praxis emancipates research by demanding inclusive, democratic, and liberatory practices. Researchers strive to see communities and participants through the eyes of a child, curious and unassuming. In this space of not-knowing, creativity is released, and space is held to invite change in the research plan and process. Cultural humility is centered when working with/in communities. Researchers question their assumptions and knowledge and surrender to the process and the possibility of unknown outcomes. This promises collective enquiry and shared power by encouraging researchers and participants, held as equals, to question rather than assume. Critical reflection ensures that prior knowledge does not get in the way of new opportunities to learn. Salt-of-the-earth researchers get comfortable with being uncomfortable and graciously hold that space for the collective to learn, adapt, and grow. Openness, trust, and co-creation flavors sustainable research and social change motivating individuals to engage in sustainable activism and social change through emergent innovative research praxis, community collaboration, and transparent data collection/analysis. Research in community art therapy projects create a wonderful stew with a recipe that is always changing and evolving as it reflects the collective efforts of the community, individuals, and researchers in understanding new knowledge, facilitating opportunities for creative action to create lasting community and social change.

Conclusion

In this chapter, I (Emily) described embodied approaches to research, using community art therapy research for social change, as a participatory act, and disseminated in language that is creative and accessible. Following the practice aims noted within the grounded theory of definition and practice, research in community art therapy is cultural and contextual, ethical, inclusive, interdependent, and non-hierarchical, attends to social issues, advocates for social justice, is embodied, and innovates the field. Continued research in community art therapy is necessary to further develop nuanced practice approaches as well as substantiate community research methods as an affective agent of change.

Art experience

Individual:

Create an image of yourself as you feel embodied.

Consider:

What do you look like?
Who is there with you?
What supports you in feeling embodied?
How do you know you are fully connected and attuned?

Community:

Create an image of what it is like to do community embodied research.

Consider:

What materials would the community use?
What does an embodied community look like?
What does the process of research look like when the community actively participates in co-regulation and the production of knowledge?
What is the salt, earth, praxis, intention, and motivation of this research?

References

Abrams, R., & Nolan, E. (2016). Developing a master's student's research and practitioner skills through collaboration with a doctoral researcher. *Art Therapy, 33*(1), 46–50. https://doi.org/10.1080/07421656.2016.1127615

Bennett, C. C., Anderson, L. S., Cooper, S., Hassol, L., Klein, D. C., & Rosenblum, G. (1966). *Community psychology: A report of the Boston conference on the education of psychologists for community mental health.* Boston University Press.

Black Smith, M. (2014, June 9). At the feet of a Master: What Georgette Seabrooke Powell taught me about art, activism, and the creative sisterhood. Truthout. https://truthout.org/articles/at-the-feet-of-a-master-what-georgette-seabrooke-powell-taught-me-about-art-activism-and-the-creative-sisterhood/

Brown, A. M. (2021). *Holding change: The way of emergent strategy facilitation and mediation.* Consortium Book Sales & Dist.

Erikson, B. (2021, June). Deinstitutionalization through optimism: The community mental health. *American Journal of Psychiatry.* Retrieved December 10, 2022, from https://ajp.psychiatryonline.org/doi/pdf/10.1176/appi.ajp-rj.2021.160404

Friere, P. (2012). *Pedagogy of the oppressed. 30th anniversary edition.* Continuum.

Jackson, L. (2020). *Cultural humility in art therapy: Applications for practice, research, social justice, self-care, and pedagogy.* Jessica Kingsley Publishers.

Jason, L. A., Glantsman, O., O'Brien, J. F., & Ramian, K. N. (2019). Introduction to the field of Community Psychology. In L. A. Jason, O. Glantsman, J. F. O'Brien, & K. N. Ramian (Eds.), *Introduction to Community Psychology: Becoming an agent of change.* Rebus Community.

Johnson, C. (2014). *The Praeger handbook of social justice and psychology.* Praeger.

Johnson, R. (2018). *Embodied social justice.* Routledge.

Joseph, C. (2006). Creative alliance: The healing power of art therapy. *Art Therapy, 23*(1), 30–33. https://doi.org/10.1080/07421656.2006.10129531

Juan, T. (2021). Development and participation: Whose participation? A critical analysis of the UNDP's participatory research methods. *The European Journal of Development Research, 33*(3), 459–481. https://doi.org/10.1057/s41287-020-00287-8

Kapitan, L. (2018). *Introduction to art therapy research* (2nd ed.). Routledge.

King James Bible. (2017). Online. https://www.kingjamesbibleonline.org/ (Original work published 1769)

Kloos, B., Hill, J., Thomas, E., Wandersman, A., Elias, M. J., & Dalton, J. H. (2012). *Community psychology: Linking individuals and communities.* Wadsworth.

Leavy, P. (2020). *Method meets art: Arts-based research and practice* (3rd ed.). Guilford.

McNiff, S. (2013). *Art as research: Opportunities and challenges.* Intellect.

Oetzel, J. G., Wallerstein, N., Duran, B., Sanchez-Youngman, S., Nguyen, T., Woo, K., Wang, J., Schulz, A., Kaholokula, J. K., Israel, B., & Alegria, M. (2018). Impact of Participatory health research: A test of the community-based participatory research conceptual model. *BioMed Research International, 2018*, 12. https://doi.org/10.1155/2018/7281405

Prilleltensky, I. (2001). Value-based praxis in community psychology: Moving toward Social Justice and social action. *American Journal of Community Psychology, 29*(5), 747–778. https://doi.org/10.1023/a:1010417201918

Prilleltensky, I., & Nelson, G. (2002). *Doing psychology critically: Making a difference in diverse settings*. Palgrave Macmillan.

Royster, R. (2021). Dolls4Peace memorial: Liberatory community art action and praxis. *Voices: A World Forum for Music Therapy, 21*(1). https://doi.org/10.15845/voices.v21i1.3153

Rubin, J. (2015). *Introduction to art therapy: Sources & resources*. Routledge.

Sarason, S. B. (1988). *The psychological sense of community: Prospects for a community psychology*. Brookline Books.

Spade, D. (2020). *Mutual aid: Building Solidarity during this crisis (and the next)*. Verso.

Stepney, S. (2019). Visionary architects of color in art therapy: Georgette Powell, Cliff Joseph, Lucille Venture, and Charles Anderson. *Art Therapy, 36*(3), 115–121. https://doi.org/10.1080/07421656.2019.1649545

Wallace, N. (2014, May 30). *The history of group art therapy with adult psychiatric patients: Semantic scholar*. unpublished thesis. https://www.semanticscholar.org/paper/The-History-of-Group-Art-Therapy-with-Adult-Wallace/6d3f5ccfc9977f50f2755461dcfa7be8dc630d5e

Zimmerman, M. (2000). Empowerment theory. In J. Rappaport & E. Seidman (Eds.), *Handbook of community psychology*. Springer. https://doi.org/10.1007/978-1-4615-4193-6_2

Chapter 8

Creative Power in Community Healing

Concluding Thoughts

Emily Goldstein Nolan

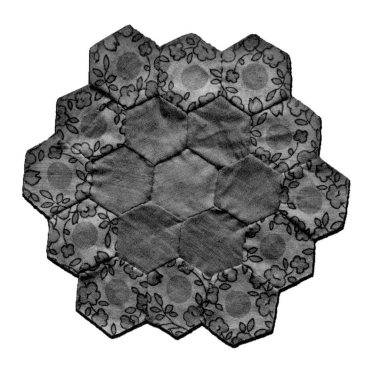

Honeycomb quilt block 8

Intrinsically, bees work cooperatively for the good of the community to create effective widescale impact and change. Bees are colony-focused and each bee's role is no more important than that of another. Bees are naturally participatory, interdependent, interconnected, highly skilled, and in tune with the ecosystem. I see that this is much like the work art therapists do in community art therapy efforts.

DOI: 10.4324/9781003193289-8

In writing this book, I set out to define community art therapy, to contribute structure to the community art therapy beehive, so to speak. As I searched for a definition, I quickly learned that I needed to challenge my own perspective of practice and include other voices and experiences. Art therapy practitioners from many different practice locales provided examples of their own work in communities, adding to the rich unfolding story of the people, places, tools, and processes using art in community healing. What emerged is a form of art therapy community guidance for those who are practicing or wish to practice in community. My vision is that anyone who reads this text finds opportunities throughout to creatively reflect on their own wisdom and ways of working in community while gathering new knowledge and validation for their own practice.

In writing this book I learned that community art therapy practitioners not only work in community settings but also approach their work with a mindset that addresses the community rather than only an individual. Their work is practiced in context and shaped by the culture of the people in that community and surrounding area, centering creative practices to both individual and collective therapeutic benefit. Community art therapy continues to grow and evolve.

I also learned that art therapy practitioners make an intention to practice skillfully and ethically. Practitioners strive to be inclusive, provide art therapy as an accessible form of healthcare and wellness practice, and facilitate spaces of true belonging. Art therapists aim to address social issues and inequities in communities, reaching beyond intrapsychic frameworks and the medical model of care to encourage interdependent, interconnected, and egalitarian relationships. Art therapists in community engage in an embodied practice of art that supports nervous system regulation.

Hopes for the Future

As I reflect on my own work in community and those experiences shared here, I am even more curious about people's experiences and stories of community art therapy efforts. I also wonder what it would be like to hear about community art therapy organizations, programs, projects, and workshops from the perspective of communities who experience creative change. I know that there are more collective voices for the whole living image of community art therapy to really come alive.

In writing this book and through talking with art therapy practitioners, I truly felt a part of a community of practice through sharing ideas, lessons learned, challenges, and resources. My dream is that everyone in the world can experience a sense of belonging and have access to the healing and transformation that artmaking with others can catalyze. I know that art therapists in social settings and using a community approach have the power to provide both.

Endnote

The quilt image for the cover and the subsequent hive quilt pieces included at the start of each chapter were from my mother. My mother is a quilter, and when I was growing up, each Wednesday after school she hosted a quilting circle at our church. Several elder women would meet there, and they would chat and sew quilts on large frames to raise money for various church projects. My mom was always on the lookout for vintage quilt tops in resale shops that they could easily place on the frame. She and I found these pieces at a resale store, and I fell in love with them. I begged her to keep them, and she did. Eventually she sewed the pieces together herself and created the quilt seen on the front cover of this book. The quilt and leftover pieces sat for years, until one Christmas while I was writing this book, my mom gave me the quilt and the pieces. This was the best present: a small reminder of the creative community that helped shape me—the hive of quilters, sewing community together.

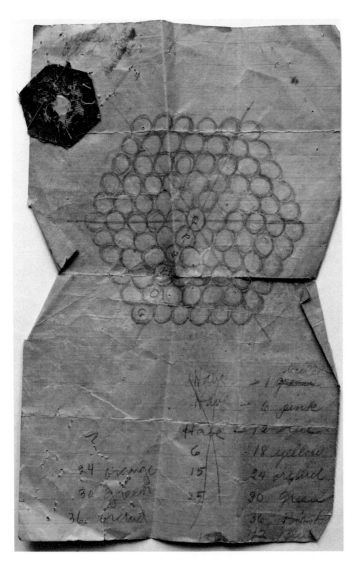

Quilt plans (front)

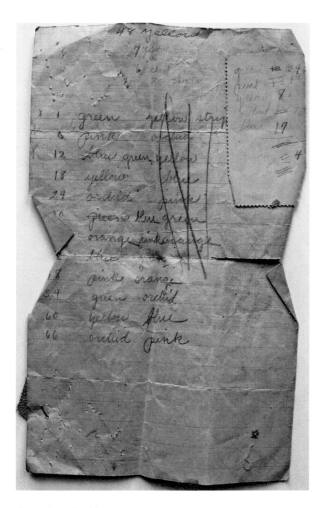

Quilt plans (back)

Index

academic language 173

Access Art Initiative 48–49, 54; access to virtual resources 50; activity centers 53; Evanston Art Connects 53; interventions 50–51; multimedia care centers 52–53; online outreach 51, 52; partnerships 49–50

accessibility 24; art material 49–50; community art therapy 16–18, 46–47; virtual resource 50

action research 153–154, 156, 161, 167–168

activism 54, 55; Black Lives Matter 85; Crafting Change 38–43; digital 61–62; LGBTQ 74–75

Adamson, G. 43

Adinkra 36

advocacy 180–182; see also activism

aesthetics 13; program development 165, 167

Albuquerque 131

Alfonso, G. 12, 25

Allen, P. 9, 115, 121

American Art Therapy Association 140, 147–148

Americans for the Arts 161, 165, 168

Animating Democracy 159, 161

anxiety 25, 85; see also trauma

approach: art therapy 11, 18; community art therapy 104; emic 58; psychosocial 21, 93

Arbeitman, E. 18

art and artmaking 12, 70; bird project 36–37; collective 26; directive 18; embodiment 24–25; healing dimension 121; hives 9, 18, 133; materials 92, 145–146; non-directive 18; silence 54–55; veteran 80–82

art museum, internship 103–105

art therapist 64, 69; bias 65; education 12; role flexibility 142–143; self-reflexivity 12; skill 15, 102; sojourner 136–140

art therapy 5, 187; approach 11; awareness 15; credentialing 111; cross-cultural 12; digital communities 59–60; ethics 15; health insurance coverage 138; in Hong Kong 45–46; innovative practice 14–15; internship 102–103; as intervention and advocacy 180–182; licensing 135; pedagogy 37–38; "pop-up" 14; practice 3, 121–122; as prevention 179, 180; regulation 15; restorative practice 109; setting 11; social justice 20; supervision 102, 109–114, 117–120, 125; training 103, 135

art-based research (ABR) 175–176

Artist Buddies 69, 70

artist identity 71–72, 121

#ArtRechargeHK 47–48

ArtStreet 131

ArtWorks 144

Asian, South Asian, and Pacific Islander (ASAPI) 52

Awais, Y. 104, 111

awareness 170; art therapy 15

Baker, S. 22, 102, 103

Bazant, M. 73

beauty queens 14

For Product Safety Concerns and Information please contact our
EU representative GPSR@taylorandfrancis.com Taylor & Francis
Verlag GmbH, Kaufingerstraße 24, 80331 München, Germany